ADOLESCENTS

IN A

MENTAL HOSPITAL

By

ERNEST HARTMANN, M.D.
BETTY ANN GLASSER, M.S.
MILTON GREENBLATT, M.D.
MAIDA H. SOLOMON, B.A., B.S.
DANIEL J. LEVINSON, Ph.D.

With the Collaboration of

Gerald Adler, M.D.
Nicholas Avery, M.D.
Harry Beskind, M.D.
Howard Corwin, M.D.
Shelley Ehrlich, M.S.

Libby Herrera, M.S.
Anton O. Kris, M.D.
Gertrude Rogers, M.D.
Bruce Sklarew, M.D.
Thalia Weiss, M.S.

Boston State Hospital

MONOGRAPH SERIES

NUMBER FOUR

GRUNE & STRATTON   New York · London

Library of Congress Catalog Card No. 67-29522

Printed in the United States of America
(C)

Contents

Part V

Outcome

Part VI

Conclusions

Part VII

Epilogue

Acknowledgments

The authors are indebted to a number of persons who advised or served the National Institute Mental Health Adolescent Research Project "Treatment of Adolescents on the Wards of a Mental Hospital," Grant No. OM-330, and have, therefore, contributed to the preparation of this monograph. Our thanks are first extended to a number of Massachusetts Mental Health Center staff members who assisted in the work of the Project but are not authors of this report; psychiatrists William Rothney, M.D., and Jay Kuten, M.D.; psychologist Lora Heims Tessman, Ph.D.; social scientists Helen Perry, Mark Spivak, Ph.D. and Carol Reiser, M.A.; social workers Adrienne Rabkin, M.S. and Ruth Goldstein, M.S. (deceased); research assistants John MacPhee and Michael Ebert.

Secretaries Rozanne Stosez, Katherine Schwager, Jean Truesdale of the Massachusetts Mental Health Center Staff; Mrs. Frances Waterman, and Mrs. Helen McGah, of the Adolescent Unit, Boston State Hospital, deserve special gratitude for their help in typing and re-typing manuscripts as do Miss Patricia Singer, Miss Margaret Hamwey, and Mrs. Evelyn Stone who served as editorial advisors, and Miss Catherine F. Hurley who provided expert financial guidance. VISTA's Eva Jo Molloy and Horst Bansner spent many afternoons proofreading the final manuscript.

We wish to thank Jack R. Ewalt, M.D., superintendent of the Massachusetts Mental Health Center, Gregory Rochlin, M.D., head of the Children's Service at the Massachusetts Mental Health Center, and William McLaughlin, M.D., superintendent of Metropolitan State Hospital who made the facilities of their respective institutions available to us, and the ladies of the Massachusetts Mental Health Center Women's Auxiliary who presented Maida H. Solomon, social work consultant to the Project, with a generous grant for a social work study of the families of the adolescent patients.

To the National Institute of Mental Health we are most grateful, for nothing that was done would have been possible without their moral support and financial aid.

Finally we acknowledge our debt to the writers and publishers of *Comprehensive Psychiatry, Journal of Health and Human Be-*

havior, and *Mental Hygiene* for their kind permission to reprint portions of the following articles:

Comprehensive Psychiatry, "Psychiatric Inpatient Treatment of Adolescents: A Review of Clinical Experiences" by Harry Beskind, M.D. Vol. III, December, 1962.

Journal of Health and Human Behavior, "The Family Structure of Hospitalized Adolescents and Their Families: A Preliminary Report" by Shelley S. Ehrlich, M.S., Vol. III, Summer, 1962.

Mental Hygiene, "The Social Adjustment of Adolescents Discharged from a Mental Hospital," by Thalia Weiss, M.S., and Betty Glasser, M.S. Volume 49, Number 3, July 1965.

Introduction

Many critics of modern society believe that something alarming is happening to adolescents both in America and in many European countries. Delinquency and crime are increasing; alcoholism and drug addiction are on the rise; impulsiveness, sexual sophistication, and acting-out are more prevalent; and hospitalization for mental illness is racing far ahead of the rate projected for the adolescent population that mushroomed as a result of the baby boom after World War II.

Almost everything has been blamed—family disintegration, divorce, affluence, poverty, sexually stimulating magazines and advertisements, deficient religious upbringing, moral decay of society, urbanization, motorization, leisure, and the threat of nuclear annihilation.

To mental health workers, the situation is especially distressing. More than ever before young people are being referred from courts, schools, and social agencies to institutional environments ill-prepared to receive them. The lack of effective programs for these adolescents struggling with critical emotional experience compounds desperation with urgency. It is imperative, therefore, that intensive investigations be undertaken in a variety of institutional settings to determine the therapeutic and non-therapeutic qualities of the environment and to plan systematic changes toward more rational and effective programs. The so-called "specific" and "non-specific" treatments for adolescents—psychotherapy, drugs, milieu therapy, etc.—need vigorous and critical study in order to evaluate their short and long-term effectiveness, yet the climate of urgency demands that innovations of any promise receive immediate field trial.

However, even if such programs within institutions should prove successful, the problem of adolescent emotional disorders would be little affected unless large-scale changes occur in society's values and youngsters' ways of socializing. Since so much of the emotional damage suffered by the adolescent is based on the change or decay of family and social organization into which he was born, the attention of mental health workers will have to encompass not only social structure but the whole span of forces and values making up our modern civilization. It goes without saying that

such a task will involve social and community psychiatric understanding of an order for which few mental health professionals are
adequately prepared. There is no escape from the fact that most of
those who have been brought up in the traditions of conventional
psychiatry will have much to learn that is new.

This is the spirit in which some six years ago we began to study
the adaptation of adolescents in a small university-affiliated hospital
that had been receiving adolescents for treatment for years, but
which had only recently begun to organize a formal program.
Adolescence had been regarded as mainly a transitional period
from childhood to adulthood which required watchful waiting. It
was now redefined as an area of specialization that might require
particular techniques and procedures. Unfortunately, because of the
paucity of clinical and research information there was very little
to guide us. Our handicaps, however, were somewhat mitigated by
the fact that for several years a study of ward and hospital organization had given us some understanding of the relevance of social
environment to patient care and treatment. An added advantage
was the fact that this hospital was committed to an intensive study
of individual psychopathology and to a therapeutic emphasis on
interpersonal dynamics.

This monograph presents the results of a multidisciplinary research experience with fifty-five adolescent patients treated on
adult wards at the Massachusetts Mental Health Center. The
adolescents were examined from the clinical, psychodynamic, developmental, and psychosocial perspective during their pre-hospital
and pre-adolescent periods, at the point of admission, during
hospitalization, upon discharge, and in several follow-up studies.

More specifically the questions we have sought to answer are:

What are the chief issues in adolescent hospital care as seen in the
literature and in other studies?
What kinds of experiences do these patients have within the hospital
that are specific to their developmental stage?
What kinds of adolescent patients are referred and admitted to a
small metropolitan teaching psychiatric hospital?
What are the effects on the other patients, the personnel and the
parents of having adolescents on adult wards?
What principal therapeutic issues arise in the treatment of hospitalized
adolescents?
To what extent are psychotherapy and other forms of treatment
used, and how successful are they?

What is the adjustment of this group at time of discharge, and later? What are the results of hospitalization?
Which adolescents achieve successful adaptation in terms of clinical outcome? Which ones fail? What variables in the pre-hospital background, at time of admission, and during hospitalization prove to be predictors of outcome?
On the basis of these studies, what kinds of special adolescent programs appear needed to treat adolescents better on various kinds of wards?

In the course of our investigations we have gained new respect for the sensitivity of these patients, for the magnitude of the task set before them in growing from childhood to maturity, and for the complexity of influences playing upon their lives. They have been rightfully referred to as "barometers of our times." Within the hospital they reflect very acutely the ups and downs of ward life; they react with large amplitude swings to the tensions and sufferings of people around them, and when they are in the community, they demonstrate this same sensitivity in their often shaky or unstable adjustment to family, school, and community.

We hope that our attempts to sharpen questions and seek answers will challenge the reader to think more deeply about problems besetting this critical age group, and above all, will assist him in his own plans to bring proper support and treatment to them.

MILTON GREENBLATT
Boston, Massachusetts
August, 1966

"Life is so complicated, tragic and confused because there really are so few adults among us. Maturity is a rare jewel, beyond price in the market of men. Adolescence is not only a stage that we have lived through but a stage of life that lives on in us. We may have repressed it; we may have forgotten about its turmoil and its tumult; but let us have no illusions: we carry the scars of our youth with us, and its attitudes shape, color and mold the clay of our spirit as long as we live."

From Hope for Man
By Joshua Loth Liebman

Copyright © 1966 by
Fan Loth Liebman
Reprinted by permission
of Simon & Schuster, Inc.

PART I

Antecedent Studies

We consider a review of the literature on hospital treatment facilities for adolescents an essential preliminary to a study of adolescents on adult wards.

CHAPTER 1

Psychiatric Inpatient Treatment of Adolescents: A Review of Clinical Experience

The earliest inpatient centers for the treatment of children, the Franklin School in Philadelphia, the children's psychiatric ward at Bellevue, the Children's Institutes of Allentown State Hospital and of Kings Park State Hospital, were designed to handle behavior disorders subsequent to the encephalitis epidemic of 1919. Patients at the Franklin School, organized in 1924, were between four and fifteen years of age. It is interesting that there were not only "organic" behavioral problems among these children but also aggressive behavior problems showing no evidence of mental deficiency, brain damage, or psychosis at time of admission.

In 1924 the Children's Institute of Allentown State Hospital opened and accommodated children up to age sixteen. For the first six years the children lived on adult wards. Klopp[25] reports, "For the most part, the adult patients took a somewhat parental interest in the children. We had practically no trouble due to petting or spoiling, although we did find the children became a source of

---

This chapter is based on the work of Harry Beskind. An earlier version was published in *Comprehensive Psychiatry*, December 1962.

irritation to the adults because of their uncontrolled behavior."
Here is immediate recognition of the problem of dealing with
aggressive behavior, as well as acknowledgment that adults could
have a therapeutic effect on children.

These hospitals were attempting to come to grips with the problems of younger patients, but failed to recognize the special needs
of adolescents. This failure has also been apparent in traditional
adult wards which admit adolescents.

Residential treatment of adolescents has been approached with a
background of general theory, much intuitive feeling, but with little
information obtained from careful clinical observation. Published
reports of inpatient adolescent care were virtually nonexistent until
the last twenty-five years and remained sparse until ten years ago,
although these patients have always been admitted to psychiatric
hospitals.

In 1946, at a symposium on the inpatient treatment of psychotic
adolescents which focused on the problem of the most favorable
hospital settings or circumstances for the management and treatment of adolescents, Cameron[7] reported a two-year experience with
fifty adolescents aged thirteen to eighteen on adult wards in England. At that time, when adolescents constituted 4.3 per cent of all
admissions, he proposed that all-adolescent units be developed in
conjunction with a general psychiatric hospital and that these units
be available for adolescents providing they did not present a
chronic problem and did not have severe behavior disorders.
Cameron felt that small wards for each sex would provide the individual with attention and control as well as "therapeutic atmosphere" although the violent psychotic adolescents could not be
cared for in such a proposed unit.

Yet at the same symposium Bardon and MacKeith,[4] who presented a two-year experience with adolescents on adult wards at
"an ordinary mental hospital," saw no reason for changing the situation even though they considered this setup less than ideal.
However, they felt strongly that delinquent adolescents were not
ill in the ordinary sense and did not belong in mental hospitals.

The views of Cameron and those of Bardon and MacKeith are
representative of the two sides of the continuing debate over the
question of the proper treatment and management of adolescents.
However, there does appear to be one point on which clinicians

agree: the treatment of adolescents on children's wards is less favorable than on either all-adolescent or adult-adolescent wards.

REPORTS FROM ALL-ADOLESCENT WARDS

A number of important papers have come from the adolescent units at Bellevue Hospital (NYC) since their inception in 1937.[9, 11, 35, 53] In 1939 Curran[11] reported the one-year experience of the first all-adolescent (male) unit in the United States. It was a short-term diagnostic and therapy center, in which various group activities and individual interviews were employed. Selection of patients by the hospital was not possible because most referrals came from the courts.* Problems of aggressive behavior were very difficult and relatively refractory. Until 1948 the ward personnel had a barred area behind which they could seek protection during riots.[35] It would be hard to imagine that this state of affairs represented improvement as compared with the experience of mixed adolescent-adult wards prior to the establishment of the unit. Toolan,[52] however, specifically states that there was "marked diminution in rebellious, volatile behavior" when the female adolescents were moved from mixed wards to all-adolescent wards at Bellevue in 1950. In 1957 an open-door policy was instituted in the male and female units. Visiting hours were extended and the daily census reduced from a range of 40-50 to 20-25. It was felt that these changes, as well as the increased ratio of ward personnel to patients, contributed to the better management of aggressive behavior.[35, 53]

In 1949 Sands[46] opened an all-adolescent unit in England. He felt that mixing of "psychopaths" with neurotic and psychotic children was undesirable. In a report on 175 cases he emphasized the use of physical methods, such as electroshock, deep insulin therapy, phenothiazines, and leucotomy, and reported a 75 per cent recovery or improvement of schizophrenics at discharge, thought to be partly due to the use of these methods. However, subsequent follow-up studies,[3] cast considerable doubt on the usefulness of such

---

* Carroll and Curran[9] reported a one-year follow-up on the first 300 male court cases admitted to the Bellevue Unit. They found that the courts accepted psychiatric recommendations in 87 per cent of cases and that 67 per cent were making a good adjustment. These percentages seemed to support the value of such a residential center as compared with figures offered by child guidance clinics.

therapies. The reason for establishing an adolescent unit was the adverse effect of adults on adolescents. Nicolson[36] too said, "Above all, it is advisable to isolate the unit from adult patients as much as possible."

The experience of Henrickson and his associates at the University of Michigan[8, 20, 21, 22, 23, 24] in developing adolescent facilities included a variety of experimental situations. The initial approach was to place adolescents aged fourteen to eighteen on adult wards. He found that one-third of the beds on an adult ward could be occupied by adolescents provided specific school, activity and therapy programs were instituted. However, the marked differences between the groups led to a negative therapeutic experience, and the demands of adolescents frequently placed the staff in a difficult position. For these reasons and because of the increasing demands for adolescent psychiatric facilities, all-adolescent wards were opened in 1956 to accommodate fifteen males and ten females.

The success of these adolescent wards was a qualified one:

> "We have found that not only do adolescents experience more anxiety over psychiatric hospitalization than do other patients, but that living on an all-adolescent ward is even more frightening to them than being on an adult ward. This seems to be true especially for boys. Even so this stimulating, competitive anxiety-arousing atmosphere favored progress in therapy for *properly* selected youngsters."[23]

Henrickson felt that placement of sicker, more impulsive and older adolescents of any diagnostic category on an all-adolescent ward was not suitable. The ability to establish an effective interpersonal relationship, some degree of impulse control and evidence of past positive experiences were considered some of the basic positive selection criteria for candidacy on an all-adolescent ward.[23] Therapy among these carefully-selected patients was flexible as to method, and was modified in relation to individual ego strengths. Psychotherapy was oriented to dealing with events of daily life. An important aspect of the milieu was a rigid social standard of conformity which tended to have a corrective effect on deviant behavior by arousing anxiety. The function of this type of environment was to supplement the verbal interpretation with concrete examples.

Suess and Hoshino[51] felt that to place adolescents on adult wards was not advisable because 1) disturbed adults are poor identification models, 2) adolescents lack normal "heterosexual social relationships" on an adult ward, 3) adolescent behavior would not be tolerated by adults or staff, and 4) a state hospital facility lacks a structured program for adolescents. From their two years' experience in a co-educational setting (two 10-bed units, male and female), they felt that selection of personnel, selection of patients and designation of a parent or a surrogate to be in contact with the hospital were the most important factors in treatment. Frequent conferences for the personnel as well as the structured program for them to follow contributed to reducing staff anxiety. Community facilities, particularly educational ones, were utilized wherever possible. Patients older than nineteen and those with sociopathic personality disturbances, primary mental defectives, organic behavior disorders, or severe sexual perversions were considered undesirable on the ward.

Only one published experience with an all-adolescent unit has come from a private psychiatric hospital. At the Hillside Hospital in New York[26, 49] an all-female adolescent unit was designed for intensive psychoanalytically oriented therapy of twenty highly selected patients. This census was too high for effective work and was subsequently lowered to sixteen. The majority of patients were either borderline or overtly psychotic. Initial therapy was oriented to dealing with the everyday realities of life. The number of staff and their qualifications were high. Even in the light of these favorable conditions, however, it was found necessary to modify the original selective criteria which included such items as "good premorbid personality" and "enough insight to want therapy in a psychiatric hospital."[49] Few sick adolescents met such rigid criteria, and patients were evaluated within a broader framework of family situation and therapeutic suitability. Consistent attitudes among staff toward patients, interstaff communication, and mutual support of staff members were considered cornerstones of the general therapeutic approach. When the unit was first established, the intention was to isolate it from the rest of the hospital as much as possible, but this plan "turned out to have unexpectedly negative results"[26] since not only the patients but also the staff felt isolated. Gradually the full facilities of the hospital were integrated into the adolescent program, particularly in the areas of recreation and the interchange of staff. This experience strongly suggested that adolescents who are having difficulty repressing id impulses are not helped on all-adolescent units, but do better on mixed adolescent-adult wards. The problems of patient selection, relatively small size of the units, and almost unanimous agreement that the most severely disturbed adolescents are best treated on adult wards suggest that the usefulness of all-adolescent units is limited.

REPORTS FROM ADOLESCENT-ADULT WARDS

Since the all-adolescent wards are beset by selection policies, limitations in the treatment of sicker and more aggressive patients, and the development of highly staffed ideal units, some clinicians have proposed that the adolescent-adult wards, with the development of specific programs, offer a more positive therapeutic or management approach to these same problems.

The reasons for establishing adolescent-adult wards center around the ego supportive, control and integrative functions that adult figures may have. A mixed ward environment will be part of the adolescent growth experience, whereas placing adolescents with their own age group may limit their opportunity for growth.[16] In normal living, adolescents group together but spend large parts of their time with adults with whom they have important and significant relationships. "The stability of an adult hospital setting should provide for the disorganized adolescents a favorable environment in which they could be helped."[30] An adult ward provides the opportunity to minimize the destructive influence of group formation during the early phases of treatment.[48] It provides opportunities for identification and tends to decrease gang formation and acting-out impulses.[13] "Children in psychotherapy seem to do better when they are in a milieu closely resembling the family structure. They react to such relationships with the impact of their own neurotic problems and unresolved dependency needs."[13] For adolescents to be successfully managed on adult wards there must also be specific programs which take into consideration selection of patients, ward setup, educational and adjunctive facilities, training and selection of personnel and social service facilities. Such programs have been established in recent years.

For many years adolescents were hospitalized on adult wards but with no specific program. In 1950 Perry and Levy[40] reported a fifty-nine year experience at a state hospital with two hundred seventy-three adolescents which showed that adolescents on an adult custodial ward responded very poorly to treatment. The adolescents constituted 1.9 per cent of admissions: 65 per cent were males, 35 per cent females; in terms of diagnosis, 34 per cent were schizophrenics, 20 per cent manic depressive, 13.5 per cent psychoses with mental deficiency, 10.5 per cent psychoses with psychopathic personality, 9 per cent psychoses due to convulsive disorder and other diagnostic categories. Only 18 per cent of the adolescents discharged made any type of satisfactory adjustment in contrast to 65 per cent of the adult population. Of fifty-six adolescents treated with physical therapies, only six responded favorably, in contrast to a 47 per cent successful outcome with adults. Later reports in the literature tend to confirm the relative ineffectiveness of somatic therapies in the treatment of adolescents.[3, 4] Perry and Levy concluded that unless adolescent units were established, "the outlook for recovery of hospitalized adolescents under state hospital conditions appears to be quite dim."

From 1944 to 1954, two hundred and twenty-five adolescent patients were treated at the Payne-Whitney Psychiatric Clinic.[16] Though adolescent patient days jumped from 8 per cent to 17 per cent during this time, all adolescents were admitted on a voluntary status. Educational, social and physical facilities were made available. Patients were placed on different wards according to the amount or responsibility and ego control they could assume. More than four or five adolescents in a 20-bed, mixed sex unit proved disruptive to the life of the ward in terms of aggressive and destructive behavior. The predominant problem was that adult patients tended to identify with adolescents and stimulate group rebellion or destructiveness. Sexual acting out was also a potential problem. Intensive psychotherapy in a milieu within which the patient could interact in a responsible manner was the basis for treatment. From this extended experience the authors concluded that such a program made it possible to treat adolescents in a general psychiatric hospital.

In 1957 Miller[30] reported the first three years' experience of treating adolescents on adult wards at the Menninger Hospital. He felt that "treatment of adolescents requires a measure of firm and consistent control combined with a flexible program of activities, education and treatment." In three years twenty-four adolescents were admitted (nine schizophrenics and fifteen character disorders). At admission, the patients could be classified in one of the following groups: 1) "I'm not sick" group, bitter about being in the hospital, but responding well to control; and 2) a more disorganized, fearful group who could be supported by firm control. All the patients had poor scholastic records on admission. Though schooling was not an enforced policy, community educational facilities were made available, and schooling became a "valued activity." There was a full range of social and physical activities. Specific rules for behavior in the hospital were elucidated at admission, but the goal was to appeal to internal rather than to external controls.

It took about three months before the patients "could recognize verbally that they were emotionally ill and were able to state their expectations from such treatment."[30] Adults did not appear to over-stimulate or exploit the adolescents. Adult patients who were only slightly older than the adolescents, however, tended to regress if they participated in adolescent activities. The general impression was that adolescents and adults got along well provided there was no delinquent behavior. Two-thirds of the adolescents became available for formal psychotherapy. Initial improvement of those patients diagnosed as schizophrenic was more rapid than those with characterologic disorders.

In a later report from the Menninger Hospital, Scofield[48] evaluated the first six years' experience (1953-1959) with forty-six patients—twelve schizophrenics and thirty-four characterologic disorders. Scofield was impressed that these patients generally showed the need to deny any dependence on adult authority figures. Yet at the same time, they also showed strong oral dependent needs and repeated behavior leading to dependence and self-destruction. The outline of the treatment program was to attempt to place adolescents in healthier relationships and identifications with adults, provide external control as needed, make available "realistic educational goals" as well as social and recreational facilities, and make psychotherapy available. The patients' total behavior was under the supervision of his hospital doctor. Though Miller felt that three months was needed before intensive psychotherapy could begin, Scofield intimated that the average period should be ten months. Since return to the home at this point in treatment could interfere significantly with the therapeutic process, patients remained in the hospital in psychotherapy for an additional six months, and then moved into family care homes. The hospital doctor continued in the capacity of administrator for a period of one year.

A point that has not received enough attention or investigation, but which Scofield clearly documents, is that the attitudes and expectations of staff contribute significantly to patients' behavioral responses. When the program was initiated there was significant anxiety and concern that the "experimental project" would be a detrimental clinical experience. Several steps were taken by the staff which, in fact, served to isolate the adolescents from the adults. As a result, the adults protested and exhibited considerable sibling rivalry. As the adult patients increased their protest, the staff began to lose their enthusiasm for the treatment of adolescents. The adolescents tended to develop an "anti-treatment sanctuary" and only after the adolescents were distributed among the adults did the problem resolve itself: "We have since moved rather consistently in the direction of minimizing the distinction between older and younger patients."[48] Their experience indicated that an adolescent population consisting of 15 per cent of the total group was optimum but that children under fifteen years did not belong on adult wards.

Falstein et al.[13] reported a two-year experience which revealed that adolescents can be hospitalized and treated in a general psychiatric hospital and that 15 per cent could be handled on an adult ward provided careful selection policies were instituted.

Schmiedeck[47] presented an experience from a state hospital where necessity demanded introduction of adolescents onto adult wards. Here the need for a program was recognized, but took the form of a shift of authority from staff to patient and the spontaneous formation of "family units." The adolescent's membership in such a group gave him access to a dependency role, but he also became a responsible member of an authoritarian body which exerted considerable control. The adolescents seemed to feel more comfortable in such a group .

REPORTS ON ADOLESCENTS TRANSFERRED FROM ALL-ADOLESCENT WARDS TO ADULT WARDS

Richter, Dietze and Lott[43] observed adolescent schizophrenic patients who had been sent to adult wards at a large state hospital because they were unmanageable in the children's unit. These patients showed striking response after transfer. Through detailed questionnaires and observations of adolescents, adults, and attendants, the authors listed the following factors as contributing to the marked improvement:

"Adult wards are considerably less stimulating than the wards of the children's unit. There are fewer activities, fewer diversions, and less emotional arousal or intensity in the pursuit of these activities.

Behavior of adult patients is on the whole less chaotic, regressive, and primitive than that of adolescents on their own wards.

On the adult wards the adolescent may experience a sharp decrease in rivalry for the attention or affections of the personnel. (The number of potential adolescent rivals is few, since usually only two to four adolescents are on a ward with the adult patients.)

The adolescents may have a special 'place' among patients on the adult wards and receive special attentions.

On the adult ward, the adolescent gains status as an adult.

In the children's unit, disturbed behavior is often reinforced and rewarded by the attentions of or imitations by fellow patients. On the adult wards such behavior is usually not rewarded.

On the adult ward the adolescent is more conscious of authortiy because of the age difference between himself and all the adult individuals and because both staff and patients conform to standards consistent with authority demands far more so than in the children's unit. Relatively more responsible behavior is expected from adult patients and is usually forthcoming.

Thus, on the adult ward there are more controlling forces than in the children's unit; thereby the adolescent is helped with the management of his own impulses."

It appears then, that it is possible to treat adolescents on either type of ward, although the consensus seems to favor adolescent-adult wards for many types of problems. In either setting, selection policies, staff attitudes, and a carefully developed program of activities are important in the successful management of adolescent patients.

Perhaps the chief problem in handling adolescent patients, constantly and repeatedly mentioned in these reports, is the control of aggressive and destructive behavior. Accordingly we shall consider this special problem in greater detail.

PROBLEMS IN CONTROLLING AGGRESSIVE, DESTRUCTIVE, AND "ACTING-OUT" BEHAVIOR

The ability to control aggressive and destructive behavior may determine whether any type of treatment setting for adolescents can survive. Though there is not complete agreement as to the meaning of "acting out" there is general consensus that it represents some form of communication and attempt to master conflicts.[28, 41] Understanding of this behavior is frequently an essential and crucial issue for individual psychotherapy. The problem of immediate intervention in the ward situation, however, usually resolves itself into the use of: 1) intuitive experience, 2) authoritarian approach because of anxiety aroused in the staff, 3) permissiveness because of reluctance to be authoritarian, and 4) influence of other patients.

Even Aichorn,[1] who approached the problem of aggressive boys with maximal permissiveness, suggested that these boys needed special handling. Hacker and Geleerd[18] clearly stated that granting unlimited freedom was unsuccessful and that it was important for the therapist to ally himself with authority. In so doing, the doctor helped to bring the patient's aggressive conflicts into the province of therapy. "The treatment goal for adolescents, therefore, can be briefly summarized as the attempt to reconcile the patient with the inevitable resignation to the demands of reality; and, by insisting on a realistic, relatively impersonal, basic minimum set of freedom restrictions, to develop capacity to stand some narcissistic wound in the process."[18]

Turle,[54] in organizing an all-adolescent male unit, initially employed permissiveness as one of the guiding principles in treatment. But the adolescents sensed this permissiveness as passivity. This policy led to more destructive behavior and finally to an organized rebellion. Turle felt that the rebellion was due to the high density of boys with delinquent and dissocial tendencies, and considered it potentially dangerous to have more than two or three dissocial boys on a ward of sixteen. Another contributory factor was that the staff was new and the anxiety level was high. The rebellion actually forced the staff into realistic parental roles.

Miller[31] reported an outbreak of delinquency among eight adolescents in a mixed adolescent-adult ward when the psychiatrist was temporarily permissive. The adolescents began "running the floor" with resultant impairment of communications between staff and psychiatrists, breakdown of relationships between adolescents and adult patients, and increased delinquent behavior. Miller felt that the fear of using authority accounted in part for the reluctance to treat delinquents in a hospital setting.

Hendrickson and Holmes[21] viewed acting-out behavior as unacceptable. Their basic philosophy was that the ". . . patient is able to control himself if he wishes." They developed a program that exposed the patients to a central adult attitude of "unavoidable reality." The authors state, "the setting is far less permissive than a high-security closed unit." If the patient cannot meet the demands of such a program, "deliberate transfer to a closed adult ward unit is clearly the answer."

Toolan and Nicklin[53] described an interesting experience with an open-door policy on an adolescent service troubled by a great deal of impulsive and aggressive behavior. This maneuver brought about a marked reduction in tension, along with a subsidence of aggressive and rebellious behavior. Although elopements increased on the male ward, they did not constitute a serious problem. Extended visiting hours, decrease of daily census, increased ration of ward personnel to patients, and the use of tranquillizer drugs also contributed significantly to ease of management.[35]

In the clinical experience reviewed above there appears to be general agreement that hyperaggressive adolescents cannot be handled conveniently on all-adolescent wards. A careful selection policy and/or transfer to an adult ward is frequently the most satisfactory solution.[7,21,27,51,54]

Goodrich and Boomer,[15] in a study of hyperaggressive children ages nine to ten, made an impressive contribution in developing principles of intervention from actual incidents between adults and children. After collecting two hundred and forty incidents, they were able to categorize them into four areas: (a) promoting personality change; (b) promoting ego growth; (c) supporting existing ego controls; (d) a staff member's management of himself. There were three general ways in which this was carried out: namely, preventive, supportive, and restitutive interventions. The preventive approaches appeared to be most important in early phases of therapy. The most successful strategy was to avoid threatening existing ego controls. Though this work is derived from experience with the children, the applicability of such methodology to adolescent management problems is not to be overlooked. Rinsley and Inge[44] have attempted to formulate "some basic messages . . . being transmitted between the treatment staff and patients," particularly at the time of the patient's entry to the hospital and in the initial phases of treatment. They describe the "adolescent position" as "a group of attitudes and behaviors" related to his illness, hospitalization, and treatment figures which are directed at vanquishing "treatment structure." A variety of devices used by adolescents to defeat structure are described. The need to recognize this behavior by the treatment team is emphasized in order that the adolescents can properly perceive the treatment structure and be assured of its continuance.

In the literature there are valuable reports on destructive and aggressive behavior as well as ways of managing it successfully[1, 11, 12, 13, 16, 18, 21, 27, 35, 38, 47, 50, 51, 53, 54] The most useful general approaches are based on the premises that such behavior is not acceptable and that definite policies are established for its control. These policies include selection and grouping of patients (proportion of asocial patients on a ward as well as proportion of adolescents to adults) transfer from all-adolescent to adult wards if necessary, specific expectations in terms of adolescent behavior and the selection, training and dynamic understanding of staff personnel. The need for clear communication among personnel is very important.

FOLLOW-UP RESULTS

Only a few studies have attempted to follow adolescents after hospitalization to answer a major question: which adolescents ultimately benefit most from which setting?

In 1942 Carter[10] presented a detailed three-year follow-up of seventy-eight consecutively-admitted psychotic adolescents between the ages of fourteen and eighteen who were on adult wards. These patients came mostly from the laboring class. Only 24 per cent were admitted on a voluntary basis, and they received no somatic therapies or psychotherapy. He designed his study to elucidate prognostic factors, and categorized his patients into four outcome groups: (a) complete recovery, (b) social recovery, (c) recurrent crises, and (d) mental deterioration and dementia requiring continued hospitalization or ending in death. Results will be presented and discussed below.

Using a similar rating scale, Masterson[28, 29] evaluated the outcome of one hundred and fifty-three adolescent patients admitted between 1936 and 1950. They included a variety of diagnostic groups, psychotic and non-psychotic, who had been hospitalized on mixed adolescent-adult wards where the emphasis was placed on psychotherapy. All were admitted on a voluntary status and came from at least a middle socioeconomic class. The patients were above average in intelligence and were chosen primarily because of their amenability to psychotherapy. Thus, Masterson's patients were carefully selected, in contrast to Carter's unselected group.

Annesley[3] reported on a two to five year follow-up and prognostic study from an all-adolescent unit.[46] Little psychotherapy was offered these patients, but emphasis was placed on a program that would provide therapy through social, educational and recreational facilities. Also employed were somatic therapies including insulin, electroshock therapy, drug therapy and leucotomy (rarely). Annesley employed four outcome categories which are similar to Carter's and Masterson's, but he calls them (a) recovered (no symptoms), (b) improved (residual symptoms but making adequate social adjustment and fully employed), (c) no change, and (d) worse. Table I presents the results and comparative data for significant improvement (categories a & b) of these three follow-up studies.

This table provides us with virtually all the statistical follow-up results published to date. These are small statistical experiences without "controls," and the criteria for diagnostic categories and follow-up evaluations are not strictly comparable. There are, however, striking similarities which give pause for serious reflection regarding the treatment of hospitalized adolescents. First, reports of improvement at discharge are quite different from long-term outcomes with respect to the schizophrenic disorders. This factor reveals the need to question carefully discharge or short-term follow-up results if used as the sole criterion of therapeutic effectiveness of residential treatment centers. There is little evidence of deteriora-

TABLE I

Comparative Data: Improvement in Adolescent Patients at Time of Discharge and at Follow-up

| | Author | Type of Ward | Total Number of Patients | Per Cent Significantly Improved | | |
				At Discharge	2-5 year Follow-up	5-19 year Follow-up
Schizophrenic Disorders:						
	Carter[10]	Adol.-Adult	47	—	30	—
	Masterson[28, 29]	Adol.-Adult	83	52	—	33
	Annesley[3]	All Adol.	78	76	42	—
Affective Disorders:						
	Carter	Adol.-Adult	17	—	83	—
	Masterson	Adol.-Adult	8	—	—	88
	Annesley	All Adol.	15	93	93	—
Psychoneurosis:						
	Masterson	Adol.-Adult	34	78	—	94
	Annesley	All Adol.	71	91	83	—
Psychopathic Personality:						
	Masterson	Adol.-Adult	20	45	—	55
	Annesley	All Adol.	198	59	60	—

tion in the follow-up results for the affective disorders, psychoneuroses or psychopathic disturbances.

A survey of discharge results from other studies[4, 9, 46, 47, 48, 51] reveals that most authors have approximately the same experience. Generally 65-75 per cent of patients show symptomatic improvement at time of discharge regardless of diagnostic category or therapeutic approach.

With reference to the magic number of two-thirds improvement at discharge, the experience of the Franklin School with aggressive children who demonstrated no organicity, intellectual impairment or psyhcoses should be cited. Morris et al.[33] reported a twenty-year follow-up on these ninety children aged four to fifteen at time of admission. They were able to follow sixty-eight to age eighteen, fifty-nine to age twenty-five, and forty-eight to age thirty or older. Their results indicated that "if the adjustment one year after observation is considered, the results would be excellent." At the time of discharge 66 per cent of the children "showed considerable improvement in their behavior." At the time of follow-up, however, only 21 per cent had made adequate social adjustment. "Contrasting this figure (66 per cent) with the latter finding of 21 per cent demonstrates how misleading immediate results can be when attempting to predict the permanent value of treatment."[33]

Second, and more important, though these three reports represent different treatment approaches during hospitalization (ranging from custodial care, physical therapies, to intensive psychotherapy), the similarity of follow-up results for all diagnostic categories suggest that the differential effect of various treatment modalities was not critical in the long-term course of the illness.

DISCUSSION

It is clear that the debate on the use of all-adolescent versus adolescent-adult wards cannot yet be resolved on any sound theoretical ground. But from the review of published empirical experience there is strong agreement that sicker adolescents are better handled on adult wards. Even though the adults are sick, they offer ego support and control not available within the peer group of the adolescents. Furthermore, although reasons for the treatment of better compensated adolescents on all-adolescent wards have been offered, there is no evidence to indicate that their experience on adult wards under proper conditions of patient selection and environment would be negative.

Beckett et al.[5] at the Lafayette Clinic attempted to assess their experiences with adolescents on a special service for boys as well as with adolescents admitted to the adult service and treated as part of the adult program in order to determine which treatment program leads to a better outcome. Average follow-up after discharge was two years, with a range of one to four years. This study could not draw definite conclusions regarding relationship between type of management and outcome; however, the follow-up results suggested that an all-adolescent service may be more helpful than a traditional adult service without a specific program for adolescents.

Certainly this debate is an outgrowth of changing attitudes toward the hospital treatment of mental patients with emphasis on the therapeutic community. This approach, in general, may indicate a trend towards mixed wards of adolescents and adults. As Redl[42] points out, however, we have no clinical assessment of the relevance of items that constitute milieu in the treatment of children.

The need for a study of selected and paired groups who have been carefully matched for known prognostic factors[3, 10, 28, 29] is indicated in order to clarify the relevance of psychiatric management and treatment procedures in the care of the adolescent.

Our impression from the literature is that adolescent-adult wards are probably preferable to all-adolescent wards for the treatment of an unselected group of adolescent patients, but there has been little thorough study of adolescents in the adolescent-adult setting.

BIBLIOGRAPHY

1. Aichorn, A.: *Wayward Youth*, New York, Viking Press. Inc. 1935.
2. Affeldt, T. O.; A survey of in-patient programs for adolescents. *Mental Hosp.* 14:208, 1963.
3. Annesley, P. T.: Psychiatric illness in adolescence: Presentation and prognosis. *J. Ment. Sci.*, 107:268, 1961.
4. Bardon, D. T., and MacKeith, S. A.: Symposium on in-patient treatment of psychotic adolescents, II. *Brit. J. Med. Psychol.* 23:110, 1950.
5. Beckett, P., Pearson, C. and Rubin, E.: A follow-up study comparing two approaches to the in-patient treatment of adolescent boys. *J. Nerv. & Ment. Dis.* 134:330, 1962.
6. Cameron, K.: Group approach to in-patient adolescent. *Amer. J. Psychia.* 109:657, 1952.
7. Cameron, K.: Symposium on the in-patient treatment of psychotic adolescents, I. *Brit. J. Med. Psychol.* 23:107, 1950.
8. Carek, D. J., Hendrickson, W., and Holmes, D. J.: Delinquency addiction in parents. *Arch. Gen. Psychiat.* 4:357, 1961.
9. Carroll, Helen M., and Curran F. J.: A follow-up study of 300 court cases from the adolescent ward of Bellevue Hospital. *Mental Hygiene* 24:621, 1940.
10. Carter, B. A.: Prognostic factors of adolescent psychoses." *J. Ment. Sci.* 88:31, 1942.
11. Curran, F. J.: Organization of a ward for adolescent in Bellevue Psychiatric Hospital *am. J. Psych.* 95:1365, 1939.
12. Edwalds, R. Konstantin, D., Tourlentes, T., and Price, J.: A state hospital's successful adolescent unit, *Mental Hosp.* 13:160161, 1962.
13. Falstein, E. I., Feinstein, S. L., and Cohen, W. P.: An integrated adolescent care program in a general psychiatric hospital. *Am. J. Ortho.* 30:276, 1960.
14. French, E. L.: Residential treatment for emotionally disturbed young people. *Mental Hosp.* 14:386, 1963.
15. Goodrich, W. D., and Boomer, D. S.: Some concepts about therapeutic interventions with hyperaggressive children, I and II. *Social Casework,* 39 1-207, II-286, 1958.

16. Greaves, D. C., Regan, P. F. III.: Psychotherapy of adolescents at intensive hospital treatment level. *In* Balsher, B. J. (Ed.): *Psychotherapy of the Adolescent,* New York, International Universities Press, 1957.

17. Green, S. Kwalwasser, S., and Stahle, A.: The role of the psychiatrist in a residential treatment unit for adolescents. *Psychiat. Quart.* (Suppl.) 34, 1960.

18. Hacker, F. J., and Geleerd, E. R.: Freedom and authority in adolescence. *Am. J. Ortho.* 15:621, 1945.

19. Hamilton, D. M., McKinley, R. A., Moorehead, H., and Wall, J. H.: Results of mental hospital treatment of troubled youth. *Amer. J. Psychiat.* 117:811, 1961.

20. Hendrickson, W. J.; Adolescent Service, Neuropsychiatric Institute, University of Michigan. *Bull. Michigan Society for Mental Health* 13:1; 1957.

21. Hendrickson, N. J., Holmes, D. J.: Control of behavior as a crucial factor in intensive psychiatric treatment in an all-adolescent ward. *Amer. J. Psychiat.* 115:969, 1959.

22. Hendrickson, W. J., and Holmes, D. J.: Planning treatment of adolescents. *Proc. Soc. Wk. Prog. Inst.* University of Michigan, 1958.

23. Hendrickson, W. J., Holmes, D. J., and Waggoner, R. W.: Psychotherapy of the hospitalized adolescent. *Amer. J. Psychiat.* 116:527, 1959.

24. Holmes, D. J.: *The Adolescent in Psychotherapy,* Boston, Little, Brown & Co., 1964.

25. Klopp, H. I.: The Children's Institute of the Allentown State Hospital. *Amer. J. Psychiat.* 11:1107, 1932.

26. Kwalwasser, S., and Green, S. L.: Treatment program at the Israel Strauss Pavilion for Adolescent Girls." *J. Hillside Hosp.* 9:14, 1960.

27. Levitt, M. and Rubenstein, B. O.: Acting out in adolescence—A study in communications. *Amer. J. Ortho.* 29:622, 1959.

28. Masterson, J. F.: Prognosis in adolescent disorders, *Amer. J. Psychiat.* 114-1097, 1958.

29. Masterson, J. F.: Prognosis in adolescent disorders-Schizophrenia. *J. Nerv. Ment. Dis.* 124:219, 1956.

30. Miller, D. H.: The treatment of adolescent in an adult Hospital—A preliminary report. *Bull. Menninger Clin.* 21:189, 1957.

31. Miller D. H.: The etiology of an outbreak of delinquency in a group of hospitalized adolescents. *In* Greenblatt, M., Levinson, D. J., and Williams, R. H. (Eds.): *The Patient and the Mental Hospital,* Glencoe, Ill., The Free Press, 1957, p. 427.

32. Moorhead, H. H. and McKinley, R. A.: Hospital management of adolescent patients. *New York J. Med.* 62:1977, 1962.

33. Morris, H. H. Escoli, P. J., and Wexler, R.: Aggressive behavior disorders of childhood. A follow-up study. *Amer. J. Psychiat.* 112:991, 1956.

34. McAtee, O. H. B., and Zirkle, G. A.: Mentally disturbed children on wards with adult mental patients. *Amer. J. Psychiat.* 116:172, 1959.

35. Nicklin, G., and Toolan, J. M.: Twenty-year follow-up of an adolescent service in a psychiatric hospital." *Psychiatric Quart. (Suppl.)* 33:301, 1959.

36. Nicolaou, G. T.: State hospital adolescent treatment unit. *Psychiat. Quart.* 30:450, 1956.
37. Noshpitz, J. D.: Notes on the theory of residential treatment. Nat. Inst. Mental Health 1958.
38. Offer, D., and Barglow, P.: Adolescent and young self-mutilation incidents in a general psychiatric hospital. *Arch. Gen. Psychiat.* 3:2, 1960.
39. Palton, R. E., and Weinstein, A. S.: First admission to New York Civil State Mental Hospital 1911-1958. *Psychiatric Quart. (Suppl.)* 34:1245, 1960.
40. Perry, H. A., and Levy, S.: The juvenile patient in the state hospital. *Dis. Nervous System* 11:111, 1950.
41. Rafferty, F. T.: Day treatment of adolescents. *In* Masserman J. (Ed.) *Current Psychiatric Therapies, Vol. I,* New York, Grune & Stratton, 1961, p. 43.
42. Redl, F.: The concept of a 'therapeutic milieu.' *Amer. J. Ortho.* 29:721, 1959.
43. Richter, M. W., Dietze, C. J. and Lott, W.: Treatment of adolescent schizophrenia and acute turmoil patient on adult wards in a state hospital. Unpublished.
44. Rinsley, D. B. and Inge, G. D.: Psychiatric hospital treatment of adolescents. *Bull. Menninger Clin.* 25:249, 1961.
45. Robinson, L. D.: Personal communication, March 1961.
46. Sands, D. E.: A special mental hospital unit for the treatment of psychosis and neurosis in juveniles. *J. Ment. Sci.* 99:123, 1953.
47. Schmiedeck, R.: A treatment program for adolescents on an adult ward. *Bull. Menninger Clin.* 25:241, 1961.
48. Scofield, J. B.: Adolescent treatment in an adult hospital. *Am. J. Orthopsychiat.* 32:660, 1962.
49. Stahl, A. S.: The first five years of the Israel Strauss Adolescent Pavilion Program. *J. Hillside Hosp.* 9:5, 1960.
50. Straight, B. and Werkman, S. L.: Control problems in group therapy with aggressive adolescent boys in a mental hospital. *Amer. J. Psychiat.* 114:998, 1958.
51. Suess, J. F., and Hoshino, A.: Therapeutic development and management of an adolescent unit in a state hospital. *Amer. J. Psychiat.* 117:891, 1961.
52. Toolan, J. M.: Female adolescent service in a psychiatric hospital. *Psychiatric Quart.* 29:239, 1955.
53. Toolan, J. M., and Nicklin, G.: Open-door policy on an adolescent service in a psychiatric hospital. *Amer. J. Psychiat.* 115:790, 1959.
54. Turle, G. C.: On opening an adolescent unit. *J. Ment. Sci.* 106:1320, 1960.
55. Warren, W.: Inpatient treatment of adolescents with psychological illness. *Lancet* 1:147, 1952.
56. Warren, W.: Treatment of youths with behavior disorders in psychiatric hospital. *Brit. J. Delinquency.* 3:234, 1953.

PART II

The Patients and the Hospital

Our study deals with a group of fifty-five adolescent boys and girls admitted consecutively during a two-year period to the Adolescent Unit of the Massachusetts Mental Health Center, a small teaching and research state hospital. These patients formed a very diversified group on admission in terms of onset of illness, diagnosis, views of self, and the manner in which they handled their drives and external threats. On the wards, the adolescents formed their own society. They were an active, impulsive group, and crises such as fights, sexual activity, running away, and suicide attempts were almost everyday events.

CHAPTER 2

Characteristics of the Fifty-Five Adolescent Patients and Their Families

THE SETTING

Adolescents have always been admitted to the adult wards of the Massachusetts Mental Health Center, but it was not until 1958 that an Adolescent Service was established as a separate admin-

Based on the work of Bruce Sklarew, Howard Corwin, and a paper entitled "The Family Structure of fifty-five Adolescents" by Betty Glasser, Shelley Ehrlich, Libby Herrera and Thalia Weiss. A preliminary report of this paper, by Shelley S. Ehrlich was published in the 1962 summer issue of the *Journal of Health and Human Behavior*.

istrative unit with Dr. Gertrude Rogers as its first administrator. The adolescent service is closely related to the children's service; senior personnel have responsibilities for both divisions. Much of the titular responsibility for the coordination of services to adolescents is assumed by the designated director of the adolescent service. However, during the three year period of our research project, there were four different part-time administrative directors, and administrative lines of authority were not fully clarified.

Massachusetts Mental Health Center is an urban teaching hospital for relatively short-term treatment. There are no custodial facilities. If a patient needs hospitalization for more than a year or two or if he is considered unmanageable on the open wards, he is usually transferred to another hospital, often to a larger state hospital.

The treatment setting here is characterized by a high staff-patient ratio, an open-door policy, emphasis on voluntary admissions as opposed to legal commitment, a lively research atmosphere, an active teaching program and a treatment philosophy concentrated on psychotherapy, but including milieu and somatic therapies.

The Center has six wards—two male wards, two female wards and two mixed wards—each providing for twenty-five to thirty patients, and a Day Hospital with about fifty patients. Adolescents are distributed about four to each in-patient service and four to the day hospital. The overall pace at the hospital is active; admissions run to eight and nine hundred a year, including thirty to forty adolescents.

The six wards and the day hospital are organized administratively under four chiefs of service who in turn are responsible to the senior echelon of the hospital. The hospital is well staffed with senior psychiatrists, psychiatric residents, nurses, attendants, psychiatric social workers, occupational therapists, psychologists, rehabilitation counsellors, as well as students in all of these disciplines. Psychiatric residents take responsibility for cases in rotation and are supervised by the chief of service and by specifically assigned senior training staff members who give intensive supervision for all cases taken in psychotherapy.

During the first year of the Adolescent Research Project, patients were admitted in order as one of the sixteen beds assigned to adolescents became available. There was always a long waiting list.

By the second year, a new admissions policy was designed to do away with the waiting list. Third-year residents in rotation spent several hours each week in brief screening interviews with referred adolescents and their parents. The majority of the adolescents were then referred to social agencies, private hospitals, and community services such as child guidance clinics. The others were admitted within a few days to the in-patient services or to the Day Hospital.

Admission policy dictated that adolescents with a wide range of clinical problems be admitted, including patients with character disorders, schizophrenia, adolescent turmoil, and severe adjustment reactions. Only severely anti-social patients with character disorders who could not be handled on an open ward were specifically excluded.

The adult patient population represented the full range of essentially acute syndromes—schizophrenia, affective disorders, psychoneurotics, organic cases and "court cases." They ranged in age from eighteen to sixty, but the majority at the time of this study was predominantly in the twenty to thirty-five age range.

The atmosphere of the hospital is academic and stimulating with lively debate among students and teachers and much experimentation within the basic structures of learning, teaching, psychotherapy, and research. An atmosphere of change is perpetuated by the pattern of rapid patient turnover and almost complete turnover of junior staff every two years.

Sample

The primary population of our study was a group of fifty-five adolescents, ages fourteen to seventeen (hereafter referred to as the "Cohort"), admitted consecutively during a two-year period to the wards of the Massachusetts Mental Health Center. The Cohort was almost equally divided between boys and girls and racially was exclusively white. All but two of these adolescents were born during World War II (1942-1945) so that the majority (70 per cent) was, at the time of hospitalization, in the fifteen to sixteen year old age group. At time of admission all but three had been living with a parent or parents, and most were the only child in the household or had only one sibling living at home.

FAMILY STRUCTURE

The families of the Cohort were divided into the upper, upper-middle and lower-middle classes (60 per cent), and the lower class (40 per cent). Professional and white collar workers were predominant (56 per cent). More than a third of the fifty-five mothers were professionally trained, most as school teachers. The majority of the fathers had histories of almost no unemployment during the patients' lifetimes, which suggests that most of these adolescents came from homes which had at least potential financial stability.

Just under half of the families were Catholic, the remainder were divided almost equally between Protestants and Jews. All the patients and most of the parents were native-born Americans.

Seventy per cent of the adolescents came from families in which the primary parental unit had, despite various vicissitudes, remained intact. The overwhelming majority of these households were composed of the nuclear family, the parents and the siblings. Eighteen adolescents were only children or had no full siblings. Among the thirty-seven who were not only children, the patient was the oldest sibling in sixteen cases, the youngest in eleven cases, and somewhere in the middle in ten cases. Thus thirty-four of the Cohort were only children, had no full siblings or were the oldest sibling. This finding may take on additional meaning if one speculates in terms of the formulation of the disturbed child functioning as the family scapegoat. In a study by Vogel and Bell[1] of families with a disturbed child, it was found that " a particular child, the scapegoat, has become involved in tensions existing between the parents" which permitted the warring parent to work out some state of marital equilibrium. Since "the eldest child was the first one available for scapegoating, he often seems to have been assigned this role and, once assigned, has continued."

Only ten families had grandparents or other relatives living in their home. While this fact gives an accurate picture of the compact household of these families, it does not begin to suggest the dominant influence of extended family members, particularly the grandparents, in the lives of these adolescents. Twenty-eight, over

[1] Bell, N. W. and Vogel, E. F. (Eds.): The emotionally disturbed child as the family scapegoat. In: A Modern Introduction to the Family, Glencoe, Ill., The Free Press, 1960, p. 383.

half of the group, had at some time been turned over to the care of their grandparents for long periods. As the dislocations of war made the parents of present-day adolescents more dependent than usual, the influence of grandparents in these children's emotional development seems particularly strong. In a review of forty-one children[2] receiving treatment at a child psychiatry unit of a hospital, the authors note that neurotic or psychotic trends can be traced through three generations. This study sought to further understanding of the grandmother as a second maternal figure for the child who reinforces or diverges from the parent's role and as a maternal figure for the mother who shapes her attitudes and responses. It also noted an awakening interest in including the grandmother in casework interviews and psychiatric studies. In addition, nine children, seven with working mothers and two from broken homes, had, at some point before they were old enough to take care of themselves, been cared for by persons other than parents or grandparents.

Loss of mother's physical presence because of employment was high among the group. Only twenty mothers had not worked outside the home during the patient's prehospitalization lifetime. Since the Cohort were World War II babies, many of the mothers began working during the manpower shortage, while the father was away in military service. In terms of separation and loss, however, the majority of the patients had not been deprived of a continuing relationship with their mothers.

Only twenty-three of these adolescents had experienced no separation (only separations of a month or longer were noted) from the father. For the thirty-two adolescents who had experienced one or multiple separations from their fathers the reasons fell into two main categories: (1) separations due to causes outside the control of the family (military service or death of the father) (2) separations due to family disintegration (marital conflict or divorce). Unfortunately, data in the records on fathers are particularly scanty. These figures do suggest that many of these adolescents have had to cope at one time or another with the actual physical loss of the father from the home, although at admission the picture presented was that of a stable family unit containing mother and father. For

[2] LaBarre, M. B. Jessner, L. and Chasing, L.: The significance of grandmothers in the psychotherapy of children. *Amer. J. Orthopsychiat*, 30, 175-185, 1960.

example, one father, since returning from war, had been working in a city twenty-five miles from the family home. He maintained a bachelor apartment in the city and lived there during the week. On weekends he would go home where he occupied a bedroom in the attic while his wife and two sons slept in the bedrooms on the second floor.

Twenty-two patients had parents (eleven mothers and fifteen fathers) with a history of mental illness, which, of course, has many implications for disordered home environment between and during hospitalization. In four instances both parents had histories of mental illness. In addition, there were twenty-one families in which nine mothers, eight fathers, and, in four cases, both parents had suffered a serious physical illness or illnesses. Although information is lacking in the following area more frequently than in any other, as far as is known, slightly more than one-half of the group also had grandparents or siblings who were hospitalized or bedridden for more than a month (at any time during the patient's life) with serious illnesses requiring the nursing care and the attention of the patient's mother.

All but nine of the forty-nine adolescents in whom the question was investigated had suffered the loss of some significant member of the immediate or extended family through death. These deaths were most often, as would be expected, deaths of grandparents, though in seven cases the patient's father had died.

PATIENT CHARACTERISTICS

I.Q. tests are not available on all these adolescents, but estimates by the doctors who knew them best showed that most were believed to be above average in intelligence: thirty were estimated to have an I.Q. over 110, including eight with an I.Q. over 130, eleven were thought to have an I.Q. in the normal range (90-110), and four had an estimated I.Q. below 90. (an estimate was not available in ten cases). However, in terms of school performance, only four were functioning ahead of their age level, twenty-one were average, and thirty were functioning one or more years below their age level. Obviously, these adolescents were not achieving their full potential in their school work.

A survey of previous illness shows that of thirty-eight patients for whom information is available, twenty-two had a previous serious physical illness (more than two weeks) and eighteen of these required hospitalization. These physical illnesses were generally not related to the patient's psychiatric illness; in only four patients was there ever a question of organicity in the psychiatric picture. Nineteen patients had had previous psychiatric hospitalization, thirteen once only and six more than once.

Enuresis past age four was noted in seventeen of the group, and this is probably a minimal estimate, since it includes only those cases in which the therapist had specific information concerning enuresis. Soiling was rare. Temper tantrums were very frequent; twenty-six patients, or 50 per cent of those for whom information was available, had a history of temper tantrums at some time in their childhood. Similarly, a history of "overt aggression" as rated by the therapist was present in thirty-three out of fifty-two. There is no question that many members of the Cohort were actively aggressive in some way as children.

About two-thirds of the adolescents had participated very little in peer-group activity. Out of forty-five for whom this information was available, only ten were considered "at least sometimes a leader" in peer relationships. Thirteen apparently had had more than one significant relationship with a friend, eight had only one such relationship, and the other twenty-four had only casual relationships or none at all. Thus many of the group had aggressive problems at one time in their lives, but they appeared to be a lonely group, with far fewer human relationships than average.

In many ways this group was typical of adolescents who might seek admission to a psychiatric hospital or service anywhere in the Boston area, but in some ways it was definitely atypical. For instance, both the socio-economic and the estimated I.Q. level were somewhat above average. This is almost certainly due to a double selection process. The patients admitted to MMHC are, first of all, self-selected since intelligent middle or upper-class parents with some connection with local universities or hospital are more likely to seek admission to this hospital for their children, as are their family doctors or psychiatrists. Second, the criteria for admission include "a good teaching case" which implies that the patient be verbal and reasonably intelligent. This, of course, tended to load the sample in the direction indicated. There may also have been a tendency to exclude adolescents with the most serious impulsive or aggressive problems, since MMHC is an open-door hospital, but this selection factor is not as clear-cut as the others.

CHAPTER 3

Admission

ADMISSION PROCESS

Every effort was made by the hospital to insure a smooth and comfortable admission. The parents were always asked to accompany the adolescent; they were usually met at the door by a social worker who introduced them to the doctor and the nurse and obtained the admission information from them over a cup of coffee in an office furnished to resemble a living room. Nevertheless, it is clear that admission was a significant and probably a frightening experience for most of the adolescents. A few of them, a very few, actually thought of themselves as young people with a specific problem that might be helped by psychiatry. For the majority, it was rather that they were being transported to a new home, to a jail, or to a boarding school.

DIAGNOSIS

The Cohort formed a very diversified group on admission. As mentioned in Chapter 2, 35 per cent had previous psychiatric hospitalizations and the majority of these formed a sort of "chronically ill" subgroup within the Cohort. Those admitted for the first time included some acutely psychotic patients, some whose difficulties at school or with the police were the chief problem, some with problems of sexual acting out, and some in a generally dejected or withdrawn state. Two admissions were described as follows:

Paul is a sixteen year old, emaciated to the point of appearing starved. His complexion is sallow and the skin seems almost transparent. His eyes seem abnormally large in the sunken-in face. His hands are held in a fairly rigid manner with the elbows and wrists bent and the fingers touching the thumb. He talks almost not at all, refuses to walk and must be carted about in a wheel chair.

This is the first hospital admission of a sixteen year old male admitted from the Boston Juvenile Court charged with larceny. The mother said that the patient had been stealing since age nine, and since age thirteen has concentrated on stealing women's underclothes. This was first discovered when he was taken to his local doctor for examination and was found to be wearing two slips.

In terms of the admitting diagnosis, twenty-four were labeled schizophrenic, two manic depressive, six character disorder, fourteen adjustment reaction of adolescence, and nine psychoneurotic. However, we felt that these diagnoses did not provide an adequate description of the patients for a number of reasons. First of all, the diagnosis was made by the admitting doctor, usually the patient's hospital doctor; there were fifty-three doctors making the fifty-five diagnoses for this group. While such a situation provides a commendable diversity of viewpoint, it also produces an obvious lack of uniformity in diagnostic criteria. Secondly, the doctor was relatively inexperienced; in fact, the adolescent was in several cases his first patient as a psychiatric resident. A third factor which might have caused distortion in diagnosis is that the doctors were hesitant to label adolescents with a diagnosis such as schizophrenia. In addition, there is a general feeling among psychiatrists, at least at the MMHC, that the usual American Psychiatric Association diagnostic categories are poorly suited for classifying adolescent patients. Accordingly the APA diagnosis was often made in an offhand or "pro-forma" manner.

Therefore the research project devised a number of criteria that might be more meaningful prognostically than the diagnostic label and which would also help in describing the patient at admission. These criteria took the form of ratings which were made by one psychiatrist after study of the patient's record, thus increasing the uniformity of rating and insuring that whatever biases were present would be constant throughout the entire group of patients.

ONSET OF ILLNESS

First the rating psychiatrist considered such a relatively simple variable as length of present illness. The duration of illness in the Cohort varied considerably. In thirteen cases the illness was judged to be of less than one year's duration; in twenty, one to three years; in nine, three to five years; and in thirteen more than five years. Thus, most of the adolescents were judged to have been psychiatrically ill for some time.

A related question was acuteness of onset. Eleven were judged to have had an acute onset in the sense of less than one month between "health" and "full-blown illness," twenty-four had subacute onset, the process lasting one month to three years, and twenty were judged to have had a gradual onset lasting more than three years. The twenty cases in the last category, however, may be an overestimation. An onset many years before admission was generally judged as gradual, since the exact facts about the onset could often not be determined. Obviously the last two questions defined patient groups with a great deal of overlap—the adolescent with a brief duration of illness generally had an acute onset, and those with a long lasting illness had a subacute or gradual onset.

The following is an example of a severely ill girl whose illness began many years before admission and developed gradually:

> Rhoda is a seventeen and one-half year old identical twin who had made marginal adjustments throughout her life, being quiet, compliant, passive. With the death of her stepfather, a man to whom the patient was quite close and attached, she seemed unable to continue functioning. Whereupon, Rhoda, at the age of fourteen, became silent, displayed inappropriate behavior, and rocked and rocked in her chair when alone. After her mother's remarriage, Rhoda seemed unable to go to school and began to posture dramatically.

The question of precipitation is always difficult, but important, since the presence of an obvious external event precipitating the illness is usually a good prognostic sign. In our group, fifteen were judged to have experienced some external event which at least helped to precipitate the illness. Of these, three were thought to have had an external factor as a chief precipitating event, while the other twelve were thought to have "mixed" internal and external factors.

The following is an example of a fifteen year-old patient whose illness seemed to have been precipitated by the death of her grandmother but was "mixed" with internal factors:

> This is the first hospital admission of Sylvia, a fifteen year-old girl sent to the hospital by her therapist for a two-week trial period in the hope of breaking up a "school phobia" which has kept the former "A" student away from school. She was seeing the image of her dead grandmother's face on her textbook when she tried to study; she also feared going to school when "my parents are home fighting like that."

One other question was asked about the present illness: "Was it a reaction to adolescence?" This question was answered "yes" in sixteen cases; that is, it was judged that "the illness bringing the patient to the hospital was not present before puberty and appeared to be a result of the increased strength of libidinal and aggressive drives at adolescence." A middle category consisted of twenty-seven cases rated "no, but. . . ." Here "the present illness was not a result of adolescence in the previous sense, but was definitely aggravated by adolescence." The other twelve cases were rated "no—the present illness was not a result of, or greatly changed by, adolescence."

Donna is an example of a girl who seemed to be adjusting well before adolescence:

> The patient is a sixteen year old high school student with above average intelligence. She presents herself as a rebellious person, concerned with her own rights, which she felt she has not been able to obtain. In earlier years she was a docile child, always obeying her grandmother who brought her up. The patient's entering adolescence has produced a change in the relationship between her and her substitute mother (maternal grandmother). The grandmother, fearful lest the patient repeat her own daughter's mistake (becoming pregnant at age sixteen), has become increasingly rigid and controlling. The immediate precipitating stress for the present hospitalization seems to have been Donna's failure to find support and help in her dilemma, coupled with the loss of two close friends who recently moved away. She therefore made an impulsive suicidal gesture for the express purpose of "getting into a hospital."

PICTURE AT ADMISSION

In terms of the picture presented on admission, the group was categorized first according to the classic "chief complaint": in six cases the chief problem was running away from home, in five it was self-destructive acts; in six, destructive acts directed at others; in six, anti-social activities; in nine, sexual aberration; in twenty, withdrawal; three cases could not be categorized.

The patients were also classified according to what sort of role they saw themselves as taking. Eleven patients considered themselves "normal," i.e., the patient, in good contact with reality, told the staff there was nothing wrong with him, that someone else sent him to the hospital by mistake or for a variety of other reasons.

Twenty-one presented themselves as "neurotic," i.e., with anxiety or complaints of some sort about themselves; and five as rebels, seeing themselves as normal or usually supernormal and misunderstood by a defective society. Six appeared to be in a state of terror or panic; five in a withdrawn state—entirely uncommunicative or "not caring." Five of the group could not be classified on this criterion.

Frank is an example of a patient who thought of himself as "neurotic":

> The patient is a tall boy who looks ten years older than his fifteen years. At admission tried to be composed—smoking a pipe—but was obviously very frightened. He was able to speak quite frankly about his fear at being in this hospital and asked whether admitting doctor thought he was as "peculiar as the other mental patients." He complained of being very inconsistent. "My moods are constantly changing. When I'm with people my own age I feel stupid and immature. I am bashful and dumb at a dance. I don't belong to any group or anything." He stated that about a year ago he was hospitalized for a few days. At that time he had an overwhelming feeling of wanting to smash everything in sight and in a rage he overturned his bed, threw things around the room, and threatened to kill his mother.

A similar question was asked in a different way. Does the patient enter with symptoms (pathology which he, himself, notices), signs (pathology that only the doctor or others notice), or both. Thirteen patients had only symptoms; twenty-five had only signs; and seventeen had both.

The following is an example of a patient who entered the hospital with both symptoms and signs:

> Danny, a small, pale, fifteen year-old boy has severe facial acne. He walks slowly and awkwardly with a duck-footed shuffling gait. He is neatly dressed, extremely polite, and agreeable. He describes himself as "nervous" and claims he wants hospitalization for his "nervousness" and to get out of his home where his father and elderly aunt live. Danny also confided in doctor that he (Danny) is involved in a plot by intelligence-spy dogs who want to take over the world from humans.

From all these variables we can only conclude for the present that our group is a very diversified one. Later, in Part V, we shall return to these variables to test them as "prognostic factors" or predictors of outcome.

Handling of Sex and Aggression

The patients were rated as to overt handling of sex and aggression during adolescence, which usually meant during the year or two prior to admission. Twenty-six patients were rated as "inhibited" in the handling of sex (no known sexual outlets or interests); fourteen were in the "normal" range, (approximately normal outlets and interests for their age); six were rated as overactive or "acting out," four had chiefly abnormal sexual activities (homosexuality, fetishism, or transvestism); and five could not be clearly classified.

Fourteen were considered "inhibited," in the handling of aggression, nine were in the "normal range"; twenty-six were categorized as overactive or "acting out," and six could not be classified. Thus, as a whole, the group tended to be inhibited sexually but found some way of acting out aggressively. This phenomenon is especially striking in the boys, two-thirds of whom were in the single category "acting out" in their handling of aggression.

Secondary Gains

The question of secondary gain was also considered. Is the illness used by the patient in order to get love or attention, or to manipulate figures in his life, and is such a factor prominent in the genesis of the illness? Although almost every illness involved at least some minor aspects of secondary gain, this factor was considered prominent in the genesis of the illness in only nine of the fifty-five patients.

Defensive Structure

Next, on a slightly more abstract level, an attempt was made to characterize the patient's psychological make-up during the present illness and at the time of admission. Several variables were used, all dealing with defensive structures or how the patient handled his drives and external threats. Perhaps the most important of these dealt with object ties. Since one of the specific tasks of adolescence is the development of object ties—the change from earlier family ties to new adult ones—we used as a guide what Anna Freud calls "defenses against infantile object ties."[3] Following Anna Freud,

---

[3] Freud, A.: *The Ego and The Mechanism of Defense.* New York, International Universities Press, 1946.

four major categories were employed to determine how the patient handled his infantile object ties. Six of the group were judged to be in the first category: displacement of libido from the early objects, chiefly parents, to friends or other newer objects (considered the healthiest way to handle object ties). Seventeen were placed in the second category: retaining the earliest objects, usually parents, but reversing the affect—turning love into hate, suddenly becoming un-cooperative and hostile to one's parents. Another seventeen were in the third category: withdrawal of libido to the self, leading to a shy, lonely state, but also sometimes leading to megalomania (ideas of grandeur about onself). The rest of the group, fifteen, were placed in the fourth and most pathological category: a retreat or regression to earlier phases, including primitive identifications and poor ego boundaries.

The above ratings underscore the obvious point that few of our group handled the adolescent problem of object ties in a truly healthy manner. In checking these categories to see whether they were of prognostic significance (Part V), we found that this classi-fication was very useful prognostically. The first two groups proved to be much better at time of follow-up than the last two groups.

CASE STUDIES

To give the reader a focused picture of individuals which the summary of overall characteristics of the group cannot provide, we shall present throughout the course of the narrative the stories of two particular adolescents in the Cohort—one who was able to make use of the hospital experience and one who was not. In this sec-tion we shall describe the past histories of these two patients, and how they appeared at time of admission:

Patrick—This seventeen-year-old, withdrawn, phobic, and some-what depressed adolescent was the only child of Irish-American parents in their early fifties at the time of his admission.

He weighed less than five pounds at birth and had considerable feeding problems in his early months. He was described as always having been strange with people—a "lone wolf" who appeared im-mature for his age. He was reluctant to play with other children, preferring to be with his parents. Patrick had asthma from age three to sixteen, but did not have serious attacks after age ten or eleven. He was an average student until the eighth grade, although he repeated fifth grade after a family move.

Patrick's maternal grandmother took an active and forceful role in caring for him in a pampering way, dominating the household for much of Patrick's first nine years. When Patrick was eight, his grandmother suffered a stroke and lived with the family for six months. Her behavior and need for care became increasingly intolerable to his parents; they arranged for her to live with her son, and the family moved away. A series of moves followed, each one closer to Boston.

When Patrick was thirteen, his grandmother died. According to his mother he initially became hysterical but rarely talked about her. He seemed to accuse his parents of responsibility for his grandmother's death which he saw as connected to their sending her away. He dealt with the loss via rituals, conducting elaborate mock Masses with friends and buying second-hand clothing that could be cut into robes and vestments.

After his grandmother's death Patrick's need to cling to his mother became stronger. Mother and Patrick frequently went to the movies and shopped together. Mother describes herself as being very close to Patrick, spending hours listening to his conversation and dreading any threat of separation, fearing that some day he would grow up and leave her. The mother is one of two children but has not communicated with her brother for many years because of disagreement about their mother's estate. She received E.S.T. for a menopausal depression when Patrick was eight, and has continued to be intermittently depressed and angry at Patrick for the trouble he caused the family.

Father, the twelfth of thirteen children, emigrated from Ireland at twenty-six. The exact extent of his drinking was never clearly ascertained, but mother frequently complained of his urinary incontinence after drinking.

Struggles between Patrick and father arose when father demanded that he perform some household chore. Patrick delayed doing the chore and responded to father's insistent demands with temper tantrums in which he threw things across the room. Father felt that he had failed Patrick by not being close enough to him at ages five to eight when grandmother dominated and babied him: "I was not a man in my own house."

The parents date Patrick's difficulties to age fourteen when he failed two subjects in parochial high school, after which he became increasingly resistant to attending school and did poor work. He behaved like a fearful, caged animal in the school, one who could not tolerate frequent heckling and teasing by peers. Because of pressure from school authorities, his parents arranged for an outpatient diagnostic evaluation. Hospitalization was decided on because of: (1) Patrick's loud temper tantrums, in which he threw furniture and screamed to the extent that his parents were afraid they would be evicted from their apartment; 2) depression, including crying, poor eating, extensive worrying about his studies and transient suicidal ideas; and (3) his phobias about walking in the street alone or talking with strange adults or peers.

Patrick was tricked into hospital admission; his mother told him that he had an appointment merely to see a doctor at the hospital. He was extremely tense and fearful, staring in fright and responding to questions with slowed speech and short answers. He said he had a lump in his throat and felt sick. During the early weeks in the hospital he constantly thought about his mother and pleaded to leave the hospital where he felt a prisoner. He complained about his mother's compulsiveness and dread of dirt which had led her to insist that he do his chores on time. The frustration of his pleas that he be allowed to do the chores after watching a particular TV program had led to tantrums. Now he cried, promised to do all his chores, and to have no more tantrums.

He offered little spontaneous material during interviews, responding to most questions in a limited, restricted way. He appeared totally devoid of feelings, and frequently said, "I don't know," although he could acknowledge slightly angry feelings toward his parents for the way they had arranged his hospitalization. He again pleaded to be let out of the hospital and to return to school, where he would do everything that was expected of him. He felt that it might be worthwhile to talk to a psychiatrist "off and on," but that he could basically take care of his own problems because his life was well planned.

Patrick at time of admission saw the hospitalization as punishment for his temper tantrums and for not having lived up to parental expectations

Linda.—Linda entered the hospital when she was fifteen with a diagnosis of acute schizophrenic reaction. She was the oldest of four sisters, one of whom suffered from severe asthma. Linda came from a middle-class Jewish family. Her father was a scientist and was considered the "intellectual" within the family structure; her mother was clearly the less educated, more insecure, and more devalued parent. There had always been latent marital discord. Family life had revolved about the asthmatic child and mother's task had been to keep her from becoming excited or nervous for fear of provoking an asthmatic attack. To that purpose much control had been exerted over other family members. As a child Linda had retreated from her mother and passively accepted a quiet and withdrawn role in the family constellation.

During late childhood Linda remained shy and seclusive, but capable of getting along with peers in a superficially adequate manner. She remained distant from mother, and chose to enjoy with her father the more "intellectual pursuits" such as music, chess, and reading, rather than share in or imitate mother in the performance of domestic duties.

Linda's difficulties appeared to be ushered in when she was thirteen. Because mother felt unable to discuss the "facts of life" with Linda, father "took the bull by the horns" and discussed sexual matters, including intercourse, directly with her. Shortly thereafter Linda consciously began to ignore father's presence. A month following their discussion, Linda began to menstruate. A marked deterioration in her relationship with father took place, and her school work, previously always good, became poor. She developed severe feelings of self-consciousness, began to isolate herself from her peers, and began to feel as if she were "in a shell."

A year prior to admission, Linda became progressively isolated and withdrawn and was placed on the waiting list at another clinic. During the year she manifested intermittent episodes of bizarre behavior. Six months prior to admission she began to show a regressive clinging dependency on both parents, wanting to get closer and closer to mother in a child-like manner. Only mother was safe; everything else terrified her. A month prior to admission she became more frantic and admitted preoccupation over sexual thoughts concerning intercourse with her rabbi. In the week just preceding admission her behavior, affective life, and thought processes further deteriorated. She hallucinated, urinated publicly, became denudative, began to talk about being taken to a "crazy house," and elaborated a delusional system in which she felt she was being followed by Communists. She spent the night before admission preoccupied with searching the house for iodine and knives, and in this agitated state was brought to the hospital.

On admission Linda was described as dark-haired, round-faced, slightly dumpy, but physically well developed. She was awkward in carriage and appeared quite immature, neither looking very feminine nor giving the appearance of a teenager. She appeared to be a lost, bewildered, confused, and frightened child. She wandered aimlessly about, appeared restless, then sat or lay down, with hands on her stomach or genitals, occasionally making undulating sexual movements with her hips and body. Her behavior was disorganized with occasional denudative periods and intermittent urinary incontinence. She showed looseness of associations, and some press of speech which alternated with periods of mumbling or muteness. She admitted that she was overwhelmed by her feelings at times. She seemed to show variable and shifting emotional affective responses, including angry episodes, laughter, and occasional crying spells. Examination of her mental status revealed her to be clearly delusional. She though of doctors as rabbis, feared a Communist plot centered about her, and questioned her own identity. Despite this chaotic picture, she was initially able to make some contact with her therapist.

CHAPTER 4

Life on the Wards

Although the adolescents lived on the adult wards at the MMHC, they were set apart from the flow of ward activity by virtue of their belonging administratively to the Adolescent Unit with its own school, study, and recreational program, by being under study by the Adolescent Research Project, and by their preference for the company of their own peer group. The service chiefs, residents and nurses were often put into a difficult position when quick decisions were needed because the Adolescent Unit was administratively separate from the six wards which made up the Adult Inpatient Service.

For much of the day, except for the few patients who were specifically restricted, adolescents could be found anywhere in the hospital, or even outside of it, more often than on their own wards. Some adolescent patients, for instance, spent a good deal of their time in the coffee shop, or in lounges of the two newest and most attractive wards. Those adolescents living on the other wards, in fact, often complained of feeling discriminated against and inferior to their peers who were housed in the new wing, although actually the assignment to the wards is random, and patients are admitted to any service that has a bed without regard to diagnosis and severity of illness.

The constant presence of an adolescent society, drawing its members from various wards and various illnesses, was of special interest to our social science colleagues. The exact membership changed, of course, but the society was always there. Special activities were organized or invented by the members; special signs or passwords and even a special language sprang up; particular meeting places were designated and reserved for the group. The society was often snobbish and exclusive—there was rivalry for leadership, and there were clear-cut in-groups and out-groups.

Based in part on work by Howard Corwin and Michael Ebert.

The boundaries of the in-group may have looked quite fuzzy and flexible to the staff observers, but they were inexorably and painfully rigid from the point of view of the adolescent who found himself excluded. There is no question that this sort of cliquish society was supportive and perhaps even necessary to a few of the adolescents—but it was certainly painful to many who found themselves rejected by the clique. Sometimes, but not always, these feelings of rejection, so immediately present, could be dealt with in individual and group therapy.

ADOLESCENT INTERACTION ON ADULT WARDS

Probably the most significant interactions on the part of the adolescents took place within their own peer group or society. This peer group was not limited by technical membership within the Adolescent Unit and included teenage "court cases," and some who were older than the Adolescent Unit cut-off age of eighteen, but nonetheless easily recognized as adolescents. In addition, there were a large number of college-age attendants, student nurses, medical, psychology, and sociology students whose social characteristics were similar to the adolescent patients. Interaction between the adolescent patients and young staff members was a distinct and important part of the therapeutic milieu, potentially helpful to many, but extremely threatening to some. There was a great deal of reciprocal interest and identification between these groups as well as considerable sexual feeling and rivalry cutting across patient-staff lines, and several adolescents became socially involved with young staff members. In one extreme case, to the consternation of the senior staff, an attendant and a female adolescent married within a few days of the patient's discharge from the hospital.

A high ratio of personnel to patients and free access by numerous visitors is generally desirable; however, during certain times of the year in the open setting of the wards of this small hospital, traffic became heavy enough to make it impossible for attendants and nurses to see who was coming in and who was going out, or who the people coming and going were. This is partly a reflection of the many visitors from all over the world who come to MMHC, of the increase in student trainees, and of the fact that more and more patients move through the hospital at will with no restrictions.

On the other hand, when temporarily emptied of its huge student-staff population on weekends, holidays, and winter recesses, the dark silence of the long echoing corridors made the hospital a most depressing and frightening place for an impressionable adolescent. Despite the weekday hustle and bustle, and because even during the week much of the activity was student-centered, a common adolescent complaint was that of "nothing to do" and of extreme boredom. Monotony is an environmental pressure hard to assess accurately from the outside. It is not usually felt by the staff member on an eight-hour shift, even if he is not busy, because he returns to a different environment before the day is over. For a young, physically healthy and energetic person living in the hospital twenty-four hours a day, the environment is often oppressive and prison-like. The recreational and occupational activities offered by the hospital are seldom enough fully to engage the interests and expend the energies of the adolescents. Many of the young patients spent part of each day in the day room, sitting silently and staring vacantly about the room. These hours of solitude would be therapeutically justifiable if the patients were turning their energies inward and considering problems fundamental to their recovery. But often they would report that they were thinking about "nothing at all."

WARD CRISES

The course of life on the wards was frequently interrupted by major and minor ward crises. A ward crisis can be defined as any incident that jeopardizes the carrying out of the fundamental responsibility of the mental hospital: to insure the welfare of the patient and the safety of those around him. A crisis is an emergency, a threatening incident compressed in time, one that often involves violence and danger.

Because of its emergency nature, the crisis generates a high level of tension and anxiety in patients and ward nursing staff. The moment a crisis arises the nursing staff member feels he is failing to meet his professional responsibilities; he dreads the possibility that a patient might meet serious harm while he is in charge. Frequently his anxiety, tension, and agitation is communicated to the patient subtly on non-verbal levels. Casual conversation is curtailed. Communications are tense, curt, often charged with urgency.

Movement of the staff about the ward is suddenly rapid and determined. Facial expressions are tense and preoccupied. There are hushed communications between staff members. There may be violence and struggle to subdue a patient. The role of the nursing staff shifts from that of friend and companion to that of custodian and watchdog. The aspect of danger in the mental hospital environment is suddenly dramatized.

For a male, in particular, the job of attendant is usually not very satisfying in self-importance, especially since his job is subordinate to that of the femal nurse. In a crisis he may suddenly become the most important person on the scene. His performance in a ward emergency is crucial to the safety of the patients. He has the keys and the power to act; the patients are unnervingly helpless before him. He may thus unconsciously dramatize the emergency nature of a crisis to the patients.

Minor Crises

The adolescents were very impulsive, frequently handling their problems by taking action: fights, sexual activity, running away, and occasionally suicide attempts. These crises, which were everyday events, could be regarded as efforts made by inarticulate teenagers to communicate feelings of anxiety, misery, worthlessness, or helplessness directly to the ward nursing staff and doctor.

Following are four examples of minor crises that occurred within the Cohort. The first example is a frequent minor crisis in which an adolescent's anger at the impending departure of his student nurse explodes:

1. An adolescent attacks a student nurse.

Henry Watson was a severely regressed schizophrenic whose hospitalization had lasted nearly two years. Jane was a student nurse who had taken on Henry as a special patient during her affiliation at MMHC. (The student nurses prepare a case study as part of their training.) Jane made a habit of visiting Henry daily, often sitting silently with him for a half hour or more. She frequently accompanied him when he went out onto the ward, sometimes holding his hand. She made considerable efforts to encourage him to take part in activities in which he would have to interact with other people. In the course of the relationship Henry became very fond of Jane. Through her patience and kindness she came to be as much of a friend of Henry as his illness would allow. She also was an object of sexual feelings—she seemed to serve as a fantasied and idealized girl-friend, and he would ask for her when she was absent from the ward. On occasion he crooned rock-and-roll songs to her, substituting her name in the lyrics. When the affiliation was drawing to a close, Jane asked Henry if he would miss her. He replied, "I'm going to miss you a hell of a lot, baby."

Jane also had a considerable emotional investment in the relationship. She was gentle and sensitive and had tried hard to make contact with this strange, regressed boy who lived largely in a private hallucinatory world. When he responded positively, she felt rewarded and complimented and consquently engaged more feeling and enthusiasm in her efforts to help him.

The crisis occurred several days before Jane made her final departure. She had been absent from work for several days and resumed work a day later than Henry expected her to. On the morning of her return she visited Henry, apologized for the misunderstanding, and mentioned again that she would be leaving soon. Jane had been careful to warn Henry repeatedly of her final departure. That afternoon she returned and suggested a walk. Henry had considerable difficulty mobilizing himself to go and seemed frightened. On the way out he darted into the bathroom and fell prone on the floor for several minutes. Finally Henry and Jane entered the elevator and started downstairs. Henry had his face to the rear wall, and Jane was remarking on a poster tacked up before him. Suddenly Henry turned on her with anger and rage, with a strange look on his face. He sprang at Jane, pinning her against the front wall of the elevator and began to pummel her with his fists. She shielded herself by clinging to the wall and taking the blows on her arm and back. The elevator ran its course, and Jane darted out when it reached the basement. She ran to the first floor and pressed the elevator button to get back to Ward 4 (the fourth floor) and get help. When the door opened, to her horror she found that Henry had never gotten off. In terror, she bolted up the remaining three flights of stairs. Help was obtained, and Henry was put in seclusion for most of the evening, during which time he was assaultive to personnel.

The desperate effort that Jane made to return to the fourth floor rather than to seek help on nearer floors is an interesting comment on the close and independent social and administrative units that each service represent in the hospital. There had been a break in communications regarding Henry's progress since the therapist had been transferred to another service shortly before this crisis and was thus no longer able to attend morning report. Whether this crisis, generally considered an outburst of anger stemming from Henry's belief that Jane was deserting him, could have been predicted and averted is a matter of conjecture.

Looking at the crisis from the perspective of the relationship of student nurses to adolescents, what is noteworthy is the degree of mutual involvement, a direct function of their similarity of age. During an interview a month after the crisis, Jane said that the experience was still vivid and crushing, that she left the hospital "confused" and that the crisis seemed to "smash everything" for her, referring to her training experience. She felt "bad" and unhappy about her last days at the hospital. The student nurse had had sufficient academic training in psychiatry to understand Henry's outburst, but she had become so identified with the patient and had placed such emotional stock in her ability to help him that his final experssion of hatred instead of love left her totally bewildered.

2. A patient escapes.

Many adolescent crises consist of an adolescent simply walking away from the hospital at a time when staff is concerned about the possibility of his suicide or assaultiveness towards others. Hospital statistics show that escapes in the adolescent group are considerably more frequent than in the adult group.

Fifteen-year-old Danny Gordon had been in the hospital several months for severe emotional difficulties during the school year. He had developed amnesia and later a bizarre delusional system with paranoid content. He was small, odd-looking, extremely withdrawn, and compulsively neat in dress. His hair was always combed straight and flat across his forehead. He walked with an awkward gait and had no athletic capability. Incredibly tense, he frequently jumped when spoken to. He was highly intelligent, and when encouraged exhibited a refreshing wit. He was the kind of boy whose fate it is to be the continual brunt of playground jokes and taunts at school.

During the summer Danny decided, with his doctor's encouragement, to take a job in the hospital's coffee shop. He worked for several days and then quit the job suddenly. With some agitation he explained that he broke dishes and was not fast enough for his work. The coffee shop staff said that his performance was fine but that he seemed very anxious. Early the next day, Danny confided in a student nurse that he planned to walk to a suburb several miles away and then decide whether he would come back. He was angry later in the morning to find out that the nurse had told the rest of the ward staff about his plan. Nevertheless he obtained permission for the walk from his doctor and left. He did not return at the ordered time, but appeared several hours later at his own home not far from the hospital. He was brought back to the hospital by his father and restricted to the back of the ward. Late in the afternoon, although he was angry and wanted to be left alone, he confided to a student observer that he had planned to jump in front of a truck after leaving the hospital. After walking the streets for several hours he lost his nerve, however, and went home instead. Shortly after the discussion Danny came runing up in real panic and made the observer swear to tell no one about his suicidal attempt, that tremendous evils would befall him if the staff or other patients were to find out. Actually the incident had already been reported to the head nurse.

Danny confided information to both the student nurse and the student observer that he did not want transmitted to the nursing staff in general. In both cases the information was important to the welfare and therapy of the patient. His willingness to talk to the observer seemed to be related to the observer's relative lack of status and authority identity on the ward. Danny had only the vaguest notion of an observer's professional role on the ward, but did know that he was not an attendant or a nurse. In the midst of an emotional crisis which mobilized anxiety and paranoid feelings about the hospital's persecuting him, lines of communication were temporarily blocked to everyone except the observer.

3. A crisis is averted.

Many of the ward crises involving adolescents frequently are centered around petty thievery.

Henry Watson, the seventeen year-old schizophrenic already referred to, was severely regressed for a long period and remained on his bed most of the day. He had on several occasions taken other patients' belongings. On one occasion he took cigarettes and a pipe from Al Regan's drawer. Al was angry and approached Henry, saying, "Come on, I know you've got them." Henry was equally hostile and very defensive. He lay on his bed with his eyes shut, holding a leather belt that he threatened to use as a weapon, and kept repeating loudly, "Get out of here." A head nurse and the observer entered the room at this point to pacify the boys and make Henry return Al's belongings. The nurse talked to Henry in a calm but firm manner for several minutes. She inquired about his angry feelings and made it clear that the belongings must be returned. When he refused to make a move himself, he was lifted to his feet and stood sullenly while the cigarettes were removed from his pocket.

During the interaction in Henry's room, the staff-adolescent relationship was primarily a communication of authority and establishment of control. It is worthwhile to see how a potentially violent and angry scene was averted. In this incident the primary communication of authority was from the head nurse to Henry. She was successful in controlling him not because of her status on the ward but because she had worked a good deal with him and had gained his respect. Her interactions with Henry were consistently understanding but firm about rules of behavior. The second communication was the threat of psysical restraint that the observer's presence and particularly his firm grasp on his arm conveyed. Henry had tussled with attendants before, and he frequently would shy away from a forbidden activity such as touching females when an attendant moved close to him.

To interpret the communicative nature of this incident from Henry's standpoint would involve analysis of his case—why he wanted to steal and the sources of his anger. It is included here merely to show that communication from staff to patient takes place on a variety of levels often simultaneously. The simple verbal order to give up the cigarettes might have resulted in violence and physical restraint. The secondary levels of communication prevented such violence: namely, the nurse's identity in the eyes of the patient and the observer's physical contact and presence.

4. An adolescent attempts suicide.

There were no successful suicides among the adolescents, but suicidal gestures constituted frequent crises among the Cohort.

Frank Donovan was an eighteen year-old psychotic patient, a postadolescent in terms of the study, but still in the process of maturing physically. He had been suspended from his first year of college for reported homosexuality and was hospitalized later in the year. His behavior on the ward was characterized by attempts to get attention such as remaining in bed and then responding coyly when aroused. During the summer he made repeated self-destructive attempts of a less than suicidal nature which often resulted in his being assigned special nurses or being placed in seclusion. The crisis described here took place on a Sunday evening, when the ward was in a general uproar. There were several new patients, each requiring special attention. One was a strong, imposing fellow who was loud, violent, incoherent, and blatantly homosexual. Each time he broke out in violence periodically throughout the evening and had to be restrained by four attendants. He frightened the other patients very much (several insisted on having their beds moved out of his room) and made the staff intensely uneasy. A second new patient was going through alcoholic tremors and could not hold down any food.

The observer reports:

"Frank Donovan had been given permission to take walks, and on the evening in question he left the hospital around nine-thirty. He had permission to be out for half an hour. Near ten p.m. the ward nurse received a call from Frank's parents. He had called home and told them he was planning to run in front of a car. Frank was listed as absent without authority, and the police were notified. However, soon after ten, Frank walked in by himself. I met him as he was being escorted down the hall by another attendant. We began walking slowly side by side, Frank dragging his feet and staring at the floor. Then with a sudden burst, he sprang out of reach and ran down the ward. I followed on his heels, yelling for help. Before I could catch him, he put his fist through a window and began lacerating his hand. I pulled him away from the window, pinned his arms behind him, and he became passive and limp. The doctor on call came up to the ward and bandaged Frank's cuts. A half hour later Frank succeeded again in slipping out of arm reach, this time with the doctor, and smashed a second window with his other hand."

A primary communication of agitation seemed to run from the the new patients to Frank Donovan. A facet of Frank's illness was undisguised homosexual desires to which he made frequent reference in conversation. All three of the new patients had homosexual backgrounds. The sudden concentration of homosexuals on the ward was a threat to him. In particular the violent patient described above was blatant and bizarre in his homosexual expressions, offering to kiss anyone who walked by. He had made remarks to Frank such as, "Don't worry, you're just like me." Frank was very curious when this patient was being restrained or secluded. It is probable that these factors, fear of loss of control and subsequent fear of physical restraint coupled with anxiety about homosexuality, triggered Frank's self-destructive attempts. After-effects in patients who have been on the periphery of a crisis can be far-reaching, for, as illustrated by the events of this account, various communications often work in a circular fashion to create a multiplicity of incidents on the ward.

A Major Crisis

In order to investigate the chain reaction of crises, two psychiatric residents working with the Adolescent Project studied the interrelationship of two events—the death by suicide of an adult patient and a theft from the hospital coffee shop the following evening—and their effects on the adolescent population. The areas of investigation include staff communications, the relevance of these events to psychotherapy, and the general behavior of the individual adolescents.

B.G., the patient who committed suicide, was a thirty-seven-year-old white married mother of two children, a university-level teacher in sociology, hospitalized for one year. During this time she was on a ward of mixed sexes including four adolescents.

She had made three attempts at suicide prior to her present and second admission to MMHC, and she had made three suicide attempts by ingestion of pills during this admission prior to her successful attempt. She was considered to be a high-risk patient in that death by suicide seemed a definite possibility.

The patient was well known to most ward members, although she did tend to remain seclusive. Her principal friends on the ward were three adult patients, all women. Among the adolescents, her relationships were quite limited; she never discussed any adolescent patient in her therapy.

Three days before her death, her therapist reaffirmed that he would not continue therapy with her beyond a seven month period and that he would help her to make arrangements with another therapist. That night she went home for her weekend privileges, but the next day her husband felt that she was too upset and should return to the hospital. Instead of doing this, she went to her therapist's apartment, broke into it, and started going through his papers. Her therapist found her in his apartment, sent her back to the hospital by taxi, whereupon she was assigned special nurses who were continued until the time of her death. Two days later, while at lunch with her special nurse, she slipped away, locked herself in a basement lavatory, soaked a sweater in chloroform (which it is presumed she had previously cached in the hospital) and wrapped it around her face. She was found shortly after by the nurse and the day supervisor and pronounced dead by the resident on call.

The following day, the chief of this service called a meeting to discuss with the patients the death and the circumstances surrounding it. Previously at morning report all therapists attending rounds were informed of the event.

The second event, the theft in the coffee shop, occurred the next evening. At night, long after the coffee shop had closed at its usual hour, four p.m., there was a dance open to the entire hospital, on B.G.'s ward. The next morning the coffee shop door was found broken open, the cash register jimmied, and thirty-one dollars taken from the till. Not until three weeks later did Jim, an adolescent patient on another ward, confess that he and another adolescent from his ward, Dave, had committed this theft. Dave, however, never admitted complicity.

The resident researchers then conducted structured interviews with or submitted questionnaires to all the therapists of the adolescent patients plus the chief of service, the head nurse, and the occupational therapist on the two wards involved.

The residents questioned all respondents about their understanding of the crisis, their sources of information, and their analysis of any simultaneous events or trends in behavior which might be connected with it. They then attempted to discover whether any patient had attempted to communicate his intention to commit any act and how the respondents had reacted to such warnings. They probed interstaff communications and asked the respondents to recall whether they had attempted to control or modify any developing situation. Finally they asked the respondents to assess the adolescents' and adults' reactions to the crisis and offer their views about the meaning of the crisis to patients and staff.

The residents discovered that communications to therapists surrounding the B.G. suicide were excellent. Only one of the fifteen therapists was unaware of this event beyond a period of one day, and this therapist had no active connection with the ward. It appears that this event was so striking as to be communicated to the therapists on all services.

However, communications about the coffee shop theft were poor. Only nine of the fifteen therapists knew anything about it, and it was known accurately by only four. This event was less charged for the hospital in general than the suicide.

Intraservice communications were studied on Jim and Dave's ward. At this level the communications were poor in that the chief and doctors did not pay attention to information coming from nurses, attendants or occupational therapists. The morale of ancillary personnel appeared to be poorest during the period following these two events—when the tension was highest.

In assessing the relevance of these two events—the suicide and the coffee shop theft—to the psychotherapy of the individual adolescents, it is clear that the events had an impact on the adolescent population, especially those on the ward in which the events occurred. On B.G.'s ward therapists considered the suicide significant in the therapy of all four adolescents. Common to all four were the issues of control and self-destructive behavior which were aroused on an overt or covert level.

On Jim and Dave's ward, the coffee shop incident appeared to have a greater impact on the adolescent population than did the suicide. After the coffee shop theft, three adolescents on this ward went through a period of overt acting out or regression. In one patient, Tim, these took the form of psychosis; in another, escape and aggressive behavior, finally culminating in his transfer; and in Dave, himself, hypochondriacal limit-testing behavior. It is perhaps significant that except for one therapist no one on this ward discussed these two events in therapy and that neither of these events was considered significant in psychotherapy.

Having defined a crisis as an increased state of tension existing within the individual or group necessitating some intervention by staff, the investigators found that these two events clearly constituted crises, both individual and group, for the adolescents involved. Following the B.G. suicide, ward meetings were necessitated, and the meeting on Jim and Dave's service was thought to bear some relation to the coffee shop theft that evening.

The nature of the contagion of feeling about impulsivity and controls on Jim and Dave's service is evident from the following sequence of events. The ward was already quite anxious because of the activities of several patients, in particular Arnold, who acted out aggressively, and Tom, who acted out homosexually. In the days immediately following the suicide, there were several specific events which directly related to it. The coffee shop theft occurred, and the search for the stolen money precipitated further overt aggressive behavior in Tom. Arnold continued to become increasingly threatening and set some fires on the ward. Many patients had personal possessions taken. Some phonographs records were thrown out the window, a couple of radios and phonographs were taken apart and parts left exposed in such a way that they constituted a danger to the other patients. It was rumored at this time that Dave and Jim were involved in the theft.

A week later, the Chief of Service, Dr. S., held a ward meeting to discuss with the patients his concern that something was going on in the ward that was making many people anxious. He talked about the destructive behavior and theft. A lively discussion ensued, particularly centered around the theft. Jim was anxious not to be present at the meeting, but he was ordered brought in by Dr. S.

On the day of the second meeting Jim and Dave got into a fight which was related to the theft, after which Jim admitted to Dr. S. that he and Dave had stolen the money. At the meeting the patients felt that stealing on the ward was no longer a problem. Jim was told that since he had admitted the robbery, he would be held responsible for half the money stolen and half the damage done to the screen door in the coffee shop. The ward subsequently quieted down a good deal. Jim, who had become psychotic in response to his guilt, started to improve. During this time it was felt that communications and morale were at the lowest point in the year on this service.

The female patients on the service responded to these events, and to sudden admission of a large group of anxious patients, in a different way, namely by increased use of medication. There was also a considerable amount of overt anxiety, expressed fear of suicide, and two suicidal gestures resulting in an increased need for special nurses.

Although the response of the adolescent patients on the two services involved was largely dictated by their independent dynamics and pathology, it appeared that the suicide helped trigger the coffee shop theft, and that both encouraged, although they did not wholly cause, the subsequent difficulties that arose on the wards.

All these crises were sources of anxiety to patients and staff, but they can also be seen as having a positive value in that they brought to light otherwise hidden aspects of relationship and communication networks on the wards.

COURSE OF HOSPITALIZATION

The process of being admitted was perhaps the only point at which the hospital course of the fifty-five adolescents was similar. Their paths then diverged markedly; about one third of the group were in the hospital less than three months (including two patients who stayed only a few days after they or their parents experienced a change of heart), one third were in the hospital three to nine months, and one third remained as inpatients for over nine months.

Even for those who spent a considerable amount of time as inpatients there were different courses of hospitalization: twenty-five spent a majority of their "hospitalized" time as full-time patients, i.e., going to school or working in the hospital; seventeen attended school in the community or worked in the community during most of their "hospitalized" period, returning to the hospital to sleep, and eight were on a day program, spending their days in the hospital but their evenings and weekends at home. Five patients were not in the hospital long enough to be placed in any of these categories.

Of the thirty-eight patients who were in the hospital long enough to make schooling a possibility, twenty-six attended at least some classes, whereas twelve refused completely to attend. Of the ones who attended, thirteen were described as "eager" to go to school, seeking it themselves, while the other thirteen were only "willing," i.e., they would go along with whatever was offered, but without enthusiasm.

Another aspect of the milieu available to all patients, which was fairly effective, was patient government. Nine adolescents were active in government meetings and a few of these held offices. Another twelve attended government meetings but were not considered active.

Ward work, in the sense of helping the attendants maintain the decor of the ward, particularly at times of parties, holidays, or special occasions, was encouraged for all patients. About half the adolescent group was regularly active in this sort of work. Housekeeping, however, was a no-man's land, for nobody on the staff was sure who was responsible for keeping the ward clean. The patients "were supposed to" take care of their own rooms, but in practice rarely did.

The treatment program varied somewhat from year to year and from ward to ward, according to the treatment philosophy of the current administrators and the ward chiefs of service, but individual psychotherapy was always a major part of the treatment. Fourteen had an average of more than two hours per week of psychotherapy, twenty-nine had one to two hours a week, and seven had less than one hour per week on the average (exact information is not available for three adolescents). In most cases—forty-four out of fifty-three—the patient kept the same resident therapist throughout his hospital stay; about half continued to see this resident for a time after discharge.

Twenty-one patients were in group therapy led by a psychiatric resident during at least part of their hospital stay. Generally speaking, group therapy was less emphasized and more loosely organized than individual therapy. First of all, there were no requirement for the patient to take part in it, and some of the patients refused. In addition, group therapy was not offered to all the adolescents. Participation depended very much on what groups happened to be running and in need of new members. Two all-adolescent groups were started during the three-year period of this project, and a number of other groups were formed which took a few adolescent members. Each psychiatric resident was expected to lead at least one group for a year, but the choice of patients was left up to him. Some groups were passed on from resident to resident, so that there were a few stable groups, but a larger number of groups which lasted six to twelve months dissolved when the resident left the hospital.

In addition to individual and group therapy with the psychiatric residents, a number of adolescents were involved in individual and group therapy experiences of various durations with medical students, student clinical psychologists, nurses, and student nurses. The exact figures on the amount of such therapy, which resulted from the multiple teaching affiliations of the hospital, are not available to us.

The policy of the hospital was that the patient always had his "own" therapist, the psychiatric resident, but that the other therapists would not be harmful, and at times could be very helpful in bringing out facets of the patient's experience that he could not or would not reveal to his resident therapist. Usually this worked satisfactorily, although there was inevitably some friction between the various therapists, each of whom felt the patient really belonged to him. The adolescents were quite frequently involved in these conflicts since they were among the more "popular" patients. It is hard to say whether such conflicts were actually harmful or helpful on the whole, but certainly they often gave the alert psychotherapist an opportunity to point out ways in which the patient was acting in his "therapeutic family" that resembled the way he acted in his own family. One amusing aspect of these multiples activities was that at times the adolescent patient had to carry an appointment book to keep track of his engagements, and in some cases this appointment book appeared as well filled as that of his doctor.

The teaching of the hospital was that, in general, drugs were to be used only in special situations in order to make psychotherapy possible or easier in an otherwise inaccessible patient. Although both residents and senior staff appeared to share this view toward drugs, thirty-one patients in the Cohort nonetheless received medication. ("Medication" implies psychiatrically active drugs other than occasional sleeping pills or single doses of tranquilizers.) In nineteen cases the medication was one of the phenothiazines; in twelve, it was either an "anti-depressant" or a "minor tranquilizer." Of the thirty-one who received medication, eight took it for less than three months, nine for three to twelve months, eleven for over twelve months. (This information is not available in three cases.) Quite often the medication was given because of pressure from nurses and attendants to control the patient's activity or disturbing behavior, rather than for intrapsychic indications. Patients who remained in the hospital longer were more likely to receive drugs in addition to psychotherapy.

Four of the group received EST at some time during their stay in the hospital. This was in each case for a psychiatric emergency, such as violent catatonic excitement or extremely disturbed behavior that did not respond to other treatment. In no case was EST part of the treatment plan at admission.

An effort was made, although not on a systematic basis, to involve the parents of the adolescents in group therapy. Fifteen of the adolescents had one or both parents in a group at some time; one of these parent groups will be discussed in detail in Chapter 10.

The policy of the hospital was to have a social worker see both parents at admission and thereafter, where possible and indicated, on a regular basis. Actually, in fifty-one cases the social worker had at least some contact with one parent, and in twenty-seven of these cases the social worker had contact with both parents. (See Chapter 9.)

It is interesting that even after a considerable period in the hospital only a very few of the Cohort saw their experience principally as a psychiatric treatment for a particular disease or malfunction. Most viewed hospitalization as an adventure or as time spent serving a sentence at a special boarding school or jail.

CASE STUDIES (*continued*)

A more intimate and detailed view of the adolescent's experience on the ward is afforded by following the progress of Patrick and Linda, the two adolescents introduced earlier.

Patrick—During the early part of hospitalization Patrick was seen in individual psychotherapy three times a week, but was not able to deal verbally with many underlying issues because of his strong resistance, fears of exposure, and "freezing up" in sensitive areas. He put great value on prompt and effective restrictions when he was not able to control himself. He compared the consistencies of the hospital's rules and regulation to the opportunities for manipulation and the uncertainty of outcomes in the family situation.

Following a few weeks of fearfulness and relative isolation, Patrick became extremely active in many hospital activities and assumed a leadership role. He made great efforts to be liked but was described by others as being bossy and over-impressed with his importance. He had a strong work orientation in his activities and soon became president of the patient government, an assistant to the director of patient rehabilitation, directed tours of the hospital, and ran errands for numerous staff members. His work in the hospital school gradually improved, so that he became one of the best students. He presented a superficial sophistication in his polite, debonair, and pompous manner and felt proud of the hospital and his role in its activities. At first he was quite distant toward other adolescents, expressing sympathy for their difficulties, but eventually was able to see common interests. After finding himself able to socialize with staff members and patients in the hospital, he then could tolerate relationships with outside peers during weekends home. At admission he had presented himself as a "confirmed bachelor" and denied any semblance of sexual feelings. After a few weeks he developed a crush on a student nurse and eventually danced with patients and thought of the possibility of marrying some day. He was able to gain some perspective on his bossiness and pomposity on discussion with staff members and in therapy, and during the course of hospitalization he gradually became less pompous and less in need of immediate approval from staff members. He did not have temper tantrums in the hospital, and the frequency and intensity of the tantrums decreased in home visits.

He appeared to be less depressed and was less phobic about meeting strangers on the street and became capable of talking with sales people.

In the hospital he was a master of ceremonies at numerous patient performances and arranged to place himself in the limelight. He hoped to be a disc jockey, announcer, or M.C. on radio or television. He wrote a newspaper for hospital circulation that contained mostly news about himself. His activity defenses served not only to keep himself unaware of underlying anxiety but also to show himself to many people. Patrick always had a strong wish to be seen and heard to assure himself that the world was not ignoring him (his temper tantrums at home represented one way that he was assured he would be seen and attended to). He referred to himself as being a showoff and acknowledged his using this role because he hoped people would recognize and like him. He saw his primary problem when admitted to the hospital as shyness, which represented conflicts about being seen and heard. He said he overcame his shyness in the hospital where he felt accepted and praised as a separate person.

Vital to his progress was his ability to solidify aspects of his identity in relating to men. His strong receptivity allowed him to "borrow" some aspects of ego functioning and identify with masculine characteristics of his therapist, the fatherly rehabilitation chief, older patients, and many other staff members. This opportunity for multiple identification with his therapist and his being accepted as a separate individual were the most important aspects of his hospital progress. At discharge he was no longer a "confirmed bachelor" who intended to join a brotherhood but was willing to consider marriage in the future. In criticizing the church, refusing to attend Mass, and considering conversion to a Protestant denomination, he asserted himself in a rebellious way against his previous basic identification and symbiotic aspects of his relationship with his mother. With the hospital's supports he was thus able to begin to stand up to her as a separate male individual.

Linda—Linda remained in the hospital for twenty-six months. Initially, emphasis was placed on helping her gain control of her wild behavior. Treatment included intensive psychotherapy, medication, pressure by personnel, and seclusion to begin to limit her socially unacceptable behavior. The initial results were gratifying, and she transiently seemed to become integrated. Thereafter she went through a hypomanic period in which she became "high" in mood and was overly involved with other people and in many projects. This then settled into an obsessional activity in which she was always busy. Early in therapy she discussed her religious and philosophical preoccupations and gradually closed over her delusional system. She became quite dependent on the hospital and on the attendant and nursing personnel. She made good initial relationships with staff nurses, doctors, and adolescent patients, did well in the hospital school and, for a brief period, became a leader in the adolescent peer group.

After seven months of continued progress she was started on the day program, spending nights and weekends at home. However, she soon became quite withdrawn and was returned to full-time hospitalization. In this context she developed a preoccupation with "dead feelings" which basically had to do with separation issues and which remained a theme in therapy throughout her hospitalization. The "dead feelings" made her very depressed, interfered with her concentration, preoccupied her at all times, and became a reason for not doing things. They prevented her from feeling close to anybody, made her feel variously alone, detached, apart, cold, and sad. She also linked these feelings with worthlessness, guilt, and being terrible, and connected them with sexual feelings for inappropriate people.

In the second year the separation issue became the focus of therapy. She felt herself displaced as a leader in the adolescent peer group and more and more isolated from home. At father's request, she told her mother to visit less often than every day. Thereafter, she regressed into an overtly psychotic state with recurrence of her marked projection and delusional system. She never again regained her previous drive, motivation, or urge to work hard to get over her illness. Her deteriorating performance, failure to utilize hospital facilities, and increasing limit-testing behavior brought increased management problems. She did not attend school regularly and forced the staff to use restrictions against which she would then rebel. She talked about going home but seemed unable to negotiate it. She would wander about the ward, alternating between feeling "high" or feeling very depressed and bemoaning her "dead feelings." Her attempts to relate to ward personnel, patients, and the adolescent peer group became increasingly inappropriate. She became bogged down in therapy. It was at this time, about nineteen months after admission, that hospitalization no longer appeared to be helping her master her difficulties. Therapeutic efforts were then directed at helping her separate from the hospital in the hope that she might be able to continue therapy as an outpatient. However, at this time her most severe regression took place. It was as if she sought through illness to maintain her contact with the hospital. When finally faced with the imminence of separation, she underwent an acute catatonic excitement state in which she thrashed wildly about, became incoherent, wildly deluded, pushed herself to the point of physical exhaustion, and appeared completely out of contact.

The dosage of Thorazine was raised to over 2000 mg./day, and she developed an agranulocytosis and leukopenia of life-threatening proportions. Wounds inflicted during her wild flailing about became infected, fever developed, and at this point emergency electroconvulsive therapy was instituted as a life-saving measure. This interrupted the cycle, and her blood picture improved, though her communications remained extremely poor. It was in this condition that she was ultimately discharged to a large state hospital for further care and treatment.

During her hospital stay, Linda received almost every treatment available. She had individual psychotherapy with the same physician throughout her entire hospitalization. In addition, she had another physician who served as an administrator during the last nine months of her hospital stay. She was in group therapy, in occupational therapy, given pharmacotherapy intermittently, and was seen in one-month periods of "therapy" by several medical students concurrently with her regular psychotherapy. Near the end of her hospital stay, she received electroconvulsive therapy at a time when all avenues of communication and therapy had broken down and she was in danger of exhaustion and death through infection, inanition, and continued self-destructive activity.

The results of each therapy individually would be difficult to evaluate. Linda's overall hospital stay cannot be regarded as successful, since it terminated in her transfer, in serious physical and mental condition, to another state hospital. What had appeared initially to be a retreat from adolescent sexuality and giving up of parental love objects, had become an issue of separation from regressive relationships which she could not be helped to resolve during her hospital stay. She was unable to separate successfully from the family emotionally or from the hospital physically. Her delusional system remained. She had not consolidated any gains that may have been transiently apparent. She left the hospital as disorganized as when she had come, having changed from an acute to a chronic patient in the process.

PART III

Attitudes Toward Adolescents
on Adult Wards

The pros and cons of various therapeutic settings for adolescents have been argued in all corners of the world without any final resolution. At the Massachusetts Mental Health Center, treating adolescents on adult wards appears to be an accepted and satisfactory policy. What did staff, adult patients, and parents really think about this program?

CHAPTER 5

Staff Attitudes Toward Adolescents
on Adult Wards

One important question we wished to answer was how satisfactory was the policy, long in use at the MMHC, of admitting adolescents to adult wards. Our focus is on the three groups of persons closest to the adolescent—hospital staff, adult patients, and the parents of the adolescents.

This chapter presents a survey of the opinions of the one hundred and sixty-four staff members of the MMHC, and an analysis of their underlying, sometimes unconscious attitudes toward the adolescent patients.

Based on work by Ernest Hartmann.

METHOD

The population studied was composed of all staff who had been at the MMHC for at least one month and had some professional contact with the adolescent patients: forty-eight doctors, thirty-five nurses, forty-seven attendants, twenty-one student nurses, six social workers, and seven occupational therapists (Table II).

A questionnaire was sent to the total sample (164) and interviews were given to a proportional sample of about 10 per cent (15 interviews), a predetermined number being chosen at random within each professional category. (See Questionnaire I, pages 67-70.)

It was felt that the questionnaire alone, while providing a large survey or "opinion poll" and giving results amenable to statistical analysis, would be insufficient since:

1. It would only assess opinions fitting into categories predetermined by us; it would not enable the respondent to develop adequately his own framework for his opinions.
2. It could give little information on reasons, on thinking, and on how the respondent had arrived at his conclusions.
3. It could reveal little about the respondent's unconscious or not quite conscious attitudes.
4. It could tell little of the "demand characteristics" of the survey, i.e., to what extent the respondent gives answers to conform with what he believes the questioner wants or expects.
5. There is a general apathy and even mild hostility toward questionnaires, stemming partly from their impersonal quality, giving respondent little personal motivation or interest.

TABLE II

Replies Received

	Sample	Completed Replies	% Replies
Doctors	48	30	63
Nurses	35	23	66
Attendants	47	28	59
Social workers	6	2	33
Student nurses	21	14	67
Occupational therapists	7	5	71
Total	164	102	62.5

The 102 respondents included 54 males and 48 females: The mean age was 27.8 years; mean length of association with MMHC, 2.5 years.

However, the interview alone would not have served the purpose because of its inefficiency as a general opinion survey, and the difficulty of analyzing the data produced.

The interviews, taking thirty to forty-five minutes, concerned the same material as the questionnaire, but in greater depth, and with additional interest focused on relations between respondent and the adolescent patients, changes in the respondent's attitudes during or due to his work, views on adolescence in general, and the relation of respondent's own experiences to the attitudes he mentions.

The chi-square technique was used to test the significance of the relationships found on the questionnaire. No statistical techniques were applied to the interview material.

Results and Discussion

On looking over the results of the questionnaire and the interviews, we noted first that the population seems to divide itself into several groups. In the questionnaire answers, for instance, one group stood out as a strongly "pro-adolescent, pro-present-system, have-learned" group. Even defined very narrowly, the group still includes thirty-seven persons, over one-third of the population answering the questionnaire. This group, which contains a large percentage of doctors and student nurses and some of the younger nurses and attendants, approved of adolescents, wanted the same number as at present or more of them on the wards, and tended to identify with the adolescents. The members of this group turned out in the interviews to be more introspective and more willing to concede problems in their own adolescence.

About half the population most often agreed with the first group, although not on all points. A third group, containing fifteen to twenty persons, almost all nurses or attendants, was definitely "anti-adolescent, anti-present system." They felt that adolescents are disturbing to the other patients and annoying to the staff, that they would be better off on all-adolescent wards, and that one learns little from them except how to control their behavior.

Taking a closer look at some particular areas may shed light on what underlies these general opinions. From the questionnaire responses there appears to be a strong feeling that the adolescents-on-adult wards system is good for staff learning, but less certainty that the system is good for adult patients, and least certainty that it is good for the adolescents. This difficulty is echoed by the long-answer responses and by several of the interviewed respondents. One of them said, "The system is good for my learning, but that is not what's important." Obviously, although the staff members felt they were learning from the adolescents, there was some guilt about having their learning favored, possibly at the expense of the adolescents.

Only twenty respondents claimed to identify more with adolescents while twenty-five identified more with adults; however, forty-two respondents admitted to having more feeling evoked by adolescents and only four to having more feeling evoked by adults (average age of these four was fifty years). Thus there was obviously a large group that had more feeling evoked by adolescents without necesarily identifying with them. It is interesting that in response to both of these questions, in regard to identification and feelings evoked, over half the population answered, "About the same; or no difference you can generalize about." The more probing interview technique did not bear this out; from the interviews it was clear that more emotion was evoked in almost everyone by adolescent patients. The results on the questionnaire probably reflect in part a general tendency to hedge, to "stick to the midde choice," and the fact that the wording "no difference you can generalize about" is attractive since the word "generalize" may have negative overtones.

This brings up an important consideration, both on the interviews and the questionnaire, namely, the "demand characteristics" of the study, or what the respondent feels is expected. The question that arise are: "What are the 'demand characteristics'?" and "What effect do these have on responses?"

The interviews were useful in investigating these points since it was often possible to tell by tone of voice, wording, etc., whether the respondent felt his opinion was "what was wanted" or "rebellious." From the interviews and some more casual conversations, a strong impression emerged of the responses that the staff respondents felt were expected or desired by the research team. These were chiefly:

> "Adolescents are good. They should be treated on adult wards. I like them personally in spite of occasional difficult moments. I've learned a lot from them."

Some respondents who in general were guarded and did not want to say much about themselves in the interview often answered almost exactly in the phrases above (i.e., conforming to what they saw as wanted by the interviewer so as to avoid being questioned or "attacked" further). Respondents who diverged from these "demand characteristics" were often truculent in their divergent responses, showing awareness of the divergence. An interesting sidelight is that on the questionnaire about 10 per cent of the respondents erased their names which had been penciled in by the researchers to facilitate distribution; the questionnaires without names were also those containing the responses that differed most markedly from the above "demand characteristics."

The effect of these "demand characteristics" on responses was hard to evaluate quantitatively, but certainly their influence was in the direction of increasing pro-adolescent responses and responses favoring adolescents on adult wards.

More thorough study of the interviews may further illuminate some of the attitudes of the pro-adolescent majority. First of all, we know already that the adolescent patients evoked a great deal of feeling. From the interviews it turns out that the feeling most consistently present was anger. In everyone interviewed, some anger could be detected. This was sometimes conscious, but a great deal of evidence also emerged for unconscious hostility towards adolescents, especially in nurses, attendants, and social workers interviewed. This hostility was most often hidden by denial on various levels and by projection:

> "They [adolescents] are fine; everything's fine; they've easy to handle; of course *some personnel* find them hard to handle. If the doctors worked on the wards eight hours a day they'd know how it is."
> "Adolescents are very well handled here. The staff doesn't get mad at them."
> "Everyone here has a lot of tolerance. You have to have tolerance with the adolescents."
> "I sometimes suspected the adolescent of malingering, but I guess most of them are really sick."
> "*The parents* often want the adolescents to be punished. *They* feel the place is too pleasant; there are too many opportunities for sexual activity here. *Parents* feel sexual acting-out should not be encouraged by the hospital."
> "It's fine this way; of course, the *older patients* are resentful."

The impression gained was that there was also a lot of unconscious jealousy of adolescents, sometimes expressed almost directly:

"They get away with so many things here."
"The staff spoils them."

sometimes by reaction formation, the respondents expressing what seems like excessive concern for the difficulties of the adolescent. The jealousy was found mainly in respondents who had definitely stopped considering themselves adolescents. There appeared to be some feeling of bitterness about rejection by adolescents, bitterness at no longer being young, and a wish to be an adolescent again.

Among the younger respondents there was marked identification with the adolescents, often not quite consciously. This was found in student nurses, younger nurses and attendants, and some psychiatric residents. These respondents often took the part of the adolescents against the staff:

"They need a place to talk without adults."
"They are used by the older patients."
"The main thing is to make them feel human."

They also tended to see the adolescents as not so sick as other patients:

"They're not very different from adolescents outside."
"They're just like adolescents anywhere."

This may in part be explained by the actual resemblance of some normal adolescent behavior to psychotic behavior, but must in part be attributed to identification with the adolescents, i.e., unwillingness to see as mentally ill a person in whom one recognizes so much of oneself.

The identification with adolescents can also become frightening to some respondents:

"They need a schedule; they should be forced into activities."
"The loose atmosphere is bad for patients . . . nurses should wear uniforms; I hate it here; I like surgical nursing. There's more authority there; you can be close to patients without being too close."

Here there is evidence that some staff members were afraid of their own adolescent characteristics. Again, they sometimes attempted to handle this by projection:

"The adolescents are so close in age to myself. This makes it difficult *for them.*"

Thus it became clear that there were numerous undercurrents within the mainstream of attitudes favoring adolescents and the present ward system.

Concerning the core group of "anti-adolescent, anti-present-system" respondents, there is less to say. No really vehement members of this group were present in the interview sample. Our impression is that the members of this group are characterized by a need to set themselves definitely apart from the adolescents and to deny their own adolescent feelings. They tended to describe their own adolescence as "average" or "normal" and to make suggestions such as "they need more control," "the staff isn't firm enough," and "get them off the adult wards." They use denial and a certain rigidity in their thinking to avoid noticing anything adolescent in themselves. Of course the reality factors must not be forgotten, i.e., that this group consisted almost entirely of "constant-contact-personnel" who have to handle patients on the ward eight hours a day and have the most immediate responsibility for dealing with acting-out by adolescent patients.

As noted, the pattern just described was most frequent in older attendants and in some nurses. Some hostility, however, was present in almost everyone. The identification with adolescents was most marked in the student nurses, but was also seen in younger nurses, attendants, and doctors. Among the doctors interviewed there was actually a sort of pride in pointing out their own adolescent characteristics, partly a pride in having insight into themselves, perhaps, but also pride because often they too had gone through a stage of denying adolescent impulses but now felt able to accept them and yet remain adult.

A rough "health" or "ego-strength" rating was given by the experimenter to each respondent interviewed. These ratings did not correlate with the patterns of opinion on adolescents. The respondents with less "ego strength" had more difficulty handling their feelings about adolescents but did not choose a particular pattern, did not lean as a group to either overidentification or overrejection.

As far as learning from adolescent patients is concerned, it certainly seems that most respondents learned something. (Although here again it must be remembered that the "demand characteristics" strongly favored stating that one had learned something.) Although the responses were quite diverse, one could loosely group "things learned from adolescent patients" into three categories:

1) Learning about adolescent patients and how to handle them (chiefly control, management, firmness; also patience, tact, etc.).
2) Learning about mental illness and patients in general
3) Learning about oneself.

Attendants, nurses and occupational therapists tended to emphasize category 1 and to some extent 2; doctors tended to emphasize category 2 and to some extent 3 and 1; student nurses tended strongly to emphasize category 3.

On the whole, there was a good level of satisfaction among the staff about treating adolescents on adult wards; however, the majority conceded that there was certainly room for improvement in the adolescent program. Some of the staff suggestions were in particular areas; i.e., planning more activities specifically for adolescents and providing one "identification figure" who would stick with the adolescent through his experiences in hospital, court, jail, etc.

Altogether it was evident from our material that the adolescent patients played an extremely important part in the experience of all categories of staff and that the staff members' own adolescent feelings and impulses, which were evoked or recalled for them by the patients, are of great significance to the staff members whether these feelings be accepted or rejected. After all, the adolescent is a creature of primitive conflicts, childish conflicts, but with an adult body at his command; frightening, but we all contain a bit of it. How could adolescents fail to fascinate us, the "adult" but obviously still partially adolescent staff members?

Questionnaire I

Adolescent Project Questionnaire for MMHC Staff Members

1) Have you had any contact with adolescent patients on the adult wards? (including the Day Hospital) Yes ( ) No ( )
2) Do they differ markedly from the adult patients? Yes ( ) "Very slightly" or "Sometimes" ( ) No ( )
3) In what ways?

4) Do you believe adolescent patients should be treated on adult wards in a mental hospital? Yes ( ) No ( )

5) *As far as the interests of the adolescent patients themselves are concerned,* do you feel:
    a) The present arrangement is an excellent one for them.
    b) The present arrangement is adequate, but needs improvement.
    c) The present arrangement is not good, but there is probably no really good way to handle adolescent patients.
    d) The present arrangement is not good. Better arrangements could be found.

6) *As far as the interest of the adult patients are concerned,* do you feel:
    a) The present arrangement (adolescents on adult wards) is an excellent one for the adult patients.
    b) The present arrangement is adequate, but needs improvement.
    c) The present arrangement is not good, but there is probably no really good way.
    d) The present arrangement is not good. Better arrangements could be found.

7) *From the point of view of your own training and learning,* do you feel:
    a) The present arrangement (adolescents on adult wards) is an excellent one for your training and learning.
    b) The present arrangement is adequate, but needs improvement.
    c) The present arrangement is not good, but probably there is no really good way, from the point of view of your training.
    d) The present arrangement is not good. Better arrangements could be found.

8) Do you consider the adolescent patients on the wards important in your training and learning experience? Yes ( ) No ( )

8a) In what way important, or not important?

9) From the point of view of your training and learning, should there be: a) more adolescent patients on the wards.
                b) less adolescent patients on the wards.
                c) about the number actually present.

10) Have you learned anything especially from the adolescent patients that you would not have learned from other patients?
     Yes ( )   No ( )

10a) What? Please explain.

11) In general, do you
    a) Feel closer to, identify more with, the adolescent patients than the adult patients?
    b) Feel closer to, identify more with, the adult patients than the adolescent patients?
    c) About the same; or no difference you can generalize about.

12) In general, do the adolescent patients
    a) Evoke more feeling (anger, joy, fear, etc.) in you than do the adult patients?
    b) Evoke less feeling in you than do the adult patients?
    c) About the same; or no difference you can generalize about.

13) If you were running the hospital, how would you arrange the treatment and care of adolescent patients?

14) In general, do you believe there are particular views, attitudes, ways of thinking, that especially characterize adolescents?
     Yes ( )   No ( )

14a) Please explain (If "yes," what are they?)

15) Please give your age: _____ Sex:_____
    Hospital service _____ or ward _____
    What is your position at MMHC? (e.g., student nurse, first-year resident, etc.) _____
    Where have you lived most of your life? _____

16) How long have you been associated with the Massachusetts Mental Health Center? _____

17) Have you had any previous experience working with ado-
    lescents? Yes ( ) No ( )

17a) If "yes," please describe.

18) How would you describe your own adolescence (age 14-18)
    in a few words?

19) Please mention here any further thoughts you may have
    about the role of the adolescent patients in your training and
    learning.

CHAPTER 6

Attitudes of Adult Patients Toward Adolescents on Adult Wards

The adolescent patients at MMHC formed a small but highly visible minority group within the context of a predominated adult hospital population. Since adult and adolescent patients had at least no overt barriers to interpersonal contact, it seemed desirable to evaluate this arrangement by examining the attitudes of the adult patients toward the adolescents.

METHOD

The data were obtained by a single clinical interview lasting sixty to seventy-five minutes. Every patient older than twenty-five who had been admitted to a ward and had remained there for more than one month, either on a full-time or part-time basis, was contacted for an interview. The sessions were semistructured; a number of prepared questions were asked in a specific order, yet time was allotted to pursue avenues of thought and to probe for more data. Notes were taken throughout the meeting, and verbatim quotations were obtained whenever possible. The attempt in these interviews was to get beneath the bland or popular comments and tap the underlying feelings and attitudes. The patients were asked questions in six major areas in the following order:

What adolescents do you know?
How well do you know them?
What do you think causes them to get sick?
In what way can we be helpful once they come here?
What is the outlook or prognosis?
What is your overall feeling about your experience with adolescents on your ward?

No effort was made to give equal emphasis to each question. Whatever area seemed to be most productive of the respondent's "core"

Based on work by Nicholas Avery.

feelings became the focus of the interview. All questions, however, were asked of each respondent.

Because each of the three in-patient services operated quite autonomously with its own chief of service and other ward personnel, there were many differences among the services which could have affected the attitudes obtained. For example, there were different arrangements made for sleeping on the three wards, one service was more committed to a Day Care orientation, and so on. These differences were not taken into account in this study; the assumption was made that the respondents from the three services were a relatively homogeneous group and that their attitudes were not a function of the differences among the three wards.

Forty-two adult respondents met the criteria of age and time spent on the wards. Of these, thirty gave enough data to be included in the survey. Approximately 10 per cent either refused to be interviewed or were not sufficiently communicative to participate. Almost 20 per cent of the original forty-two patients started the interview but failed to complete it because of excessive anxiety, disinterest, etc. Some 71 per cent, then, of the total eligible population was used.

Of the thirty respondents who could be included, only six were males. This one-to-four ratio compared with a two-to-three male-to-female sex ratio for the entire hospital. The age range of the thirty was twenty-five to fifty years, with a mean of 31.5 years. Ten adolescents, six males and four females, were on the three services at the time of the survey, approximately evenly distributed. The age range at time of admission was fourteen to seventeen years with an average age of 15.9 years.

We analyzed the characteristics of these respondents in terms of their social and personal distance from the adolescents, their feelings about the etiology of the adolescents' illnesses, their thoughts about prognosis, and their recommendations for treatment. On this basis, the respondents were divided into "anti," "ambivalent," and "pro" adolescent groups. Of the thirty respondents, nineteen (63 per cent) had predominantly unfavorable attitudes toward the adolescent. Seven (23 per cent) were ambivalent and four (13 per cent) were favorably disposed.

SOCIAL AND PERSONAL DISTANCE

By social distance is meant a feeling on the part of the adult that the interests, activities, and social skills of the adolescents are remote from his own. The following are direct quotations which may illustrate this item:

> "I find it hard to relate to eighteen- and seventeen-year-olds. Our interests are poles apart . . . they play that blasted rock and roll until I feel like taking an axe to the machine."
> "Their social life is a hot problem. I saw A.M. with a group of boys go off into a dark corridor. Since they can't date, they flirt on the ward and mix among themselves. I've forgotten how to do that."

In terms of personal distance, the adolescents were perceived as being different with regard to various physical or personality traits. For example:

> "The younger ones just think of girls and love. I no longer think that way."
> "Mental illness is just another experience to them."
> "They have small minds."

As one might expect with such stereotyped views, there were many contardictory opinions. One such disparity was that adolescents are both very lazy and have a good deal of energy.

Sometimes social and personal distance feelings were manifested by the recommendation that the adolescents be placed on a separate ward. Thirty-nine per cent of the "anti" group approved of a separate setup; however, 11 per cent of this "anti" group saw some advantage to having the adolescents with them. The remaining 50 per cent mentioned distance feelings without specifically recommending a separate unit. For example, some were against a separate unit because they felt the adolescents would become violent or because they would monopolize the staff's time. Almost exclusively they said the advantage in living on an adult ward was to the adolescent (he would benefit from their advice, etc.). None in the "pro" or "ambivalent" groups advocated a separate ward for the adolescents. The "anti" group of respondents, in general, tended to experience greater social and personal distance from the adolescents. Most described minimal or no social interaction with them.

ETIOLOGY OF THE ADOLESCENTS' ILLNESS

Everyone in the three groups blamed something or someone when discussing the cause of mental illness in the adolescent. Parents were frequently criticized for being either too restrictive or too indulgent of the sexual and aggressive drives within their adolescent children. The "anti" group was unanimous in declaring the cause of the adolescent's illness to be sexual or aggressive excesses: too many sexual experiences too early in life, staying up too late, drinking excessively, etc. Likewise, all agreed that the adolescent was too violent, rebellious, delinquent, or assaultive or that he was too irresponsible, pampered, selfish, or shiftless.

In the "pro" and "ambivalent" groups, there were many more similarities than differences in their perceptions of cause for mental illness. These two groups, however, could be distinguished from the "anti" group. Fifty-seven per cent of the "ambivalent" respondents and all of the "pro" adult patients did not limit themselves to blaming either parent or adolescent. Instead they mentioned parental death, strong genetic influence, frustrated life goals, rejection by peer group, and the normal turbulence of adolescence as predisposing factors. In this group there was quite a bit less moralizing. Feelings of inferiority, loneliness, frustration and insecurity were identified as the affects experienced by the adolescent as he became ill. The "anti" group, on the other hand, felt that the outlawed sexual or aggressive experience *per se*, caused the illness in many cases. The following excerpts are from "anti" respondents:

> "They need a sense that their parents are their parents . . . . They get too much freedom and that leads to unhappiness. They should be told, 'In this house there are rules. If you don't want to obey the rules, get out.' Many of them start begging 'I'll be good.' The parents should say, 'No, out!' There's nothing wrong in whippings; I was spanked plenty as a child, and it didn't harm me a bit . . . the parents have these little monsters and argue with them by the hours—one slap does much more . . . these juvenile delinquents, they're treated dreadfully in court. They commit all this vandalism and destruction and the judge just laughs at them. They're put on probation, given curfews, or lose their licenses or are made to pay back for the property they destroyed. But that's all; they still get their [school] letters, or trips to Washington. I don't mean to be severe, but that's not my idea of just punishment . . . . In most things I'm tolerant; with sexual deviation I'm not in the least bit tolerant. I'm not swayed by any arguments about how many thousands do it or who's to say

what's normal or by what psychiatrists say to them. They just want an excuse, the easy way; they want people to condone them, but it'll be on their conscience for as long as they live."

This militantly moral stance, probably representing a reaction formation, colored the comments of many patients in the "anti" group. When this reaction is coupled with the autobiographical nature of the perceptions, some insight can be gained about the reasons for this disavowal of libidinal expression. This will be elaborated in the discussion section.

The next quote is from another patient and illustrates clearly the dualism in her feelings. In part she identified with the teenager and resented the parental prohibitions. However, she was also very harsh and punitive herself with regard to sexual expression. This dual attitude was naturally rationalized, i.e., only certain kinds of sexual expression were taboo. But this rationalization was quite unsubstantiated in this case:

". . . her parents brought her [E.N., an adolescent patient] here because they couldn't sit out her experimentation with emotion, awareness of herself, and sex. Parents try to keep you pure and quiet. Sometimes there's a lot of hostility toward the child from the parents. I prefer a hellion and working with raw material."

At this point she became aware that she was talking about her own life, that she wasn't allowed to rebel, that her parents were restrictive and her father a "die-hard." Having realized this, she shifted in her orientation:

"I can't stand immorality. Immoral people are the worst degraders of human nature. They should be abolished at all costs."

By immorality she meant:

". . . intercourse before wedlock, necking and petting—a healthy teenager will not pet."

Once more she changed her vantage point and assailed the restrictive forces in (?her) life.

"If a teenager is raised in church and things like that, he'll get sick too because his platonic love is inhibited."

In addition to other factors the ambivalent responses blamed the parent, the child, or both but with much less emphasis on sexuality and aggression. For example:

"They're too serious, want to get good grades too much and when they don't, they break down . . . . Mother's death, couldn't take it. . . . They feel they're not accepted by their friends, year after year . . . it affects them and they might withdraw . . . end up feeling alone without any friends."

". . . they withdraw on themselves . . . become less sociable, more concerned with themselves . . . that was my trouble too, I was too interested in myself . . . I was fearful I'd be hurt by the group. I was alone a lot . . . you forget how to make friends and end up hating yourself."

Although the blaming continued into the "pro" group, its focus and character changed noticeably. Only the parents were blamed, and the identification with the adolescent was much stronger. Completely absent was the moral indignation against the teenager for his unbridled instinctual life. The trend to mention uncontrollable factors such as parental death, which characterized the "ambivalent" group, continued:

". . . they're frustrated in their goals, . . . education, friendship, marriage, children . . . there's no distinction between an adolescent and an adult . . . can occur at any age . . . family doesn't understand them . . . it's very important to have a good family behind one . . . it's important to be able to talk to people who understand you . . . this shares the burden."

"E.B. needs a mother who understands him . . . he doesn't get much help . . . he's looking for a mother figure . . . there's a terrific amount of rejection . . . split families . . . family not interested or understanding . . . the parents are probably poorly adjusted with their own problems . . . heredity plays a role . . . adolescence is a vulnerable time anyway."

In summary, the "anti" group felt the teenager brought his problems on himself because he was reluctant to curb his impulses, but also, to a lesser extent, they blamed his parents for this lack of control. The "ambivalent" and "pro" groups were more temperate in their blame-fixing and shifted to a somewhat less moralistic position. They allied much more with the adolescent and viewed him more as a person whose needs were not met.

RECOMMENDATIONS FOR TREATMENT

The same attitudes operative in designating the causes of mental illness influenced the respondents to suggest various therapies. When sexual extremes were considered the determinants of the maladjustment, they outlined measures to suppress this behavior. If the adult picked out aggressive or violent behavior as causal items, he also tended to advocate their prompt control. The adolescent was viewed by some as out of control and disruptively nonconforming in his behavior. Accordingly, this group saw as "therapeutic" measures which would effect, *by force if necessary,* the desired amount of docility and bring the patient to a "healthy" frame of mind. Of note was the lack of concern for the adolescent's own therapeutic aims. A strong note also in this orientation was the avowed value of keeping the adolescent "busy." The proposed activity was justified on a variety of grounds but was clearly perceived by many as forestalling the devil's mischief.

These attitudes may be summarized under the heading of an authoritarian orientation. As might be expected, the "anti" group was the most authoritarian; next came the ambivalent group and least, the "pro" group, who tended to emphasize the beneficial effects of warm, friendly and supportive contacts. People were seen as more important to an adolescent than activity; further, their helpfulness was acknowledged as being *in response* to some expressed need on the teenager's part.

When asked how we can be helpful to the adolescent, this is what some "anti" respondents said:

". . . they need a social life of their own, amongst themselves . . . when they are unruly like R.C., she had temper tantrums . . . I had plenty of my own at her age . . . have to handle them firmly, I believe in firmness . . . I was badly disciplined and I suffered for it . . . give them a more regimented life instead of them floating around . . . they need strong discipline . . . our society suffers from too much freedom for children . . . I'd be very firm with them about their responsibility for rooms and for doing their ward work . . . with penalties if the rules are not abided by."

"Patients who come here should abide by the rules . . . pitch in and help because they all live here . . . lots of them figure because they're sick they're not supposed to do anything. . . . I think work is important because if they don't work around the house, they won't work outside. I tell my kids what we teach you, you will teach. We're older and we know."

The punitive and authoritarian tone became slightly muffled in the ambivalent group:

". . . the adolescent wants to feel we're interested in him as a person—talking with him, particularly engaging with him in activities . . . we also have a responsibility not to let adolescents infringe on our rights; in the ward meetings when the adolescents talk too much, I tell them to shut up very firmly . . . in showing them their transgressions, it helps them define their domain. . . ."

Least authoritarian in the proposed treatment plans were the "pro" group. However, traces of the "big stick" attitude were evident in the second of these two excerpts:

"They've got to be treated as the age they are . . . some have no sex education . . . some need a more permissive atmosphere . . . here they're pretty much accepted . . . help them come to some decisions . . . granting them permission if they bring themselves to ask . . . encourage them to see that they *are* capable . . . give them credit for effort at least. . . ."

". . . filling in the missing blanks . . . offset loss of parent . . . it's important to express feelings . . . I had no one to confide in . . . I started out asking my doctor questions, I find this helps me . . . there's enough supervision here . . . they're put on restrictions when bad and get off when good, just like an older patient . . . an adolescent's more likely to run away, restrictions help this. . . ."

A vigilant attitude, strict supervision and, above all, control were the therapeutic gestures applauded by the "anti" group. Instinctual expression was clearly taboo, and the force of authority was advocated to bear against it. Less authoritarianism and more attention to the unmet needs was characteristic of the "pro" group. The "ambivalent" group embraced elements of both extremes on the issue of therapy.

Prognosis

Surprisingly, the most optimistic group with regard to prognosis was the "anti" group; the ratio of favorable to unfavorable was 6:1. Next in order of optimism was the "pro" group with a ratio of 3:1; and, last, the "ambivalent" group with a 2:1 ratio of favorable to unfavorable outlooks. Many of the respondents spontaneously elaborated their reasons for an optimistic prognosis. The chief reason mentioned was the youth of the adolescents *per se*. Many of these respondents neglected to say whether the prognosis was good or not but posed their reply in terms of a comparison between the adolescent and adult prognoses. All but one of the respondents who made a comparison felt the adolescents had a better prognosis. The exception was a "pro" respondent.

The following quotations are from "anti" respondents who gave reasons for their optimism:

> "The doctors and nurses prefer to work with the younger ones. They're not so ingrained . . . can only go so far with adults. . . ."
> ". . . their life is not too complicated . . . they more or less have had security in their lives . . . after being sick, they can shrug off their illness . . . they don't take things as seriously as a grown-up does. . . ."
> "I think they have a better chance than me and my old ways. I've had them for thirty-seven years. . . . I'm set in my ways . . . hard for me to pull up roots."

Some reasons given by "ambivalent" patients were:

> ". . . psychotherapy would work for an adolescent because they don't think of things as much . . . they have fleeting thoughts . . . adults read . . . form their own opinions . . . they know already what's wrong."
> ". . . they can be molded or changed . . . chances are best with children, next adolescents, then adults. . . ."

The "pro" respondent who felt the prognosis might be worse for the adolescent speculated that the early illness might reflect a lower threshold for stress. The envy behind many of the responses was clearly seen in the reasons for the optimistic views. The most stereotypic thinking was in evidence in these comments. In some cases this envy emerged as a frank statement to the effect that the adolescent is "faking." Twenty-five per cent of the "ambivalent" group and twenty-six per cent of the "anti" group mentioned their distrust of the adolescents' veracity and suspected him of simulating a mental illness. No such feeling was expressed by the "pro" group. In addition, frank and open hostility was expressed by the "ambivalent" and "anti" group both toward the adolescent patient and toward the staff.

There were suggestions that the hostility was linked to feelings of envy. A great deal of anger was directed at so-called "excessive" use of recreational facilities. For instance, one patient wanted to take an axe to the record player. Anger at the staff for favoring the adolescents was evident in this quotation:

> ". . . the attendants are young and have the same interests as the adolescents . . . they go down to their level . . . they're all jazz fans

too . . . the student nurses should have a more professional attitude . . . they tend to be a bit too familiar . . . they dance and have long conversations with the patients . . . the patient might over-react. . . . I know an attendant who dated a patient. . . ."

One patient became very angry at a student nurse who sat with a regressed female patient and gently urged her to talk:

"They just sit and stare at the patient. If I were J. [the patient], I'd jump up and slap them [the student nurses]. You can't get any conversation that way. I can get her to talk: they can't. I'll say things that she'll have to answer."

DISCUSSION

The first thing that emerged from the analysis of the interviews was that the material was largely autobiographical. Many respondents broke off their account and confessed that they were really talking about themselves, their own adolescence and their parents. It mattered far less what the adolescents on the wards were like and much more what the respondents' past lives were like. The attitude expressed also served to justify the respondent's past experience. If whippings were frequent in his life, then they were deemed valuable and necessary. If a great deal of deprivation or frustration had been the respondent's lot, then overindulgence and "spoiling" a child were condemned.

It would be a mistake to view the "anti" and "pro" groups as being fundamentally opposed in their attitudes. In none of the three groups was there a sharp either/or identification with adult or adolescent. Rather, patterns of identification emerged with a seemingly predominant orientation. In the "anti" group, the focus was on identification with the parent; it was the sexual, irresponsible, or "spoiled" adolescent himself who was blamed for the illness. However, there was a good deal of hostility directed toward parents as well. This emerged obliquely, directing itself against the hospital staff and parents who indulge their children. Another popular defense against parent-directed anger was reaction formation. The anger was masked by a pious deference to parental, social, and religious authority and by a hyper-moralistic condemnation of the adolescent's sexual and aggressive urges.

The "pro" group were able to empathize much more with the younger patient and to aim their anger and blame directly against the parents. They seemed to have obtained more gratification from older figures and accordingly advocated more tolerance and support for the younger patients. Here the focus in the identification pattern was clearly with the adolescent. There also seemed to be less hostility directed at their parents, less moralizing, and much less authoritarian orientation.

The "ambivalent" group, at least within the scope of a single clinical interview, did not have a clear-cut orientation toward either adolescent or adult. For the most part their attitudes were characteristic of both the "pro" and "anti" groups. Furthermore, they indicated that a shift in the direction of empathy was related to the source of frustration. Thus, they were willing to tolerate the adolescent *provided* he didn't become obnoxious; they were also quite willing to censure his parents (or staff) and to take the adolescent's side if he seemed to merit this alliance.

CHAPTER 7

Parental Attitudes Toward the Hospital Experiences

Research social workers, following the outline of a special questionnaire, interviewed one or both parents of twenty-seven members of the Cohort, to learn of their perception of the hospital and the treatment programs. Only parents whose children had been hospitalized for at least three months were approached for interviews. In five of the thirty-six cases who qualified, the adolescents left the hospital so soon after the three months that the social workers were unable to set up research interviews, and in four cases the parents were not available. The data obtained from the questionnaire were then recorded on a pre-coded form.

One of the main purposes of this study was to find out how parental attitudes toward the hospital experience correlated with successful or unsuccessful adaptation and treatment. Another major area of interest was the attitudes of parents toward having their children housed on adult wards. Other questions concerned the parents' feelings about having their child hospitalized, the actual admission process, special difficulties during the first months, specific hospital polices such as open wards, non-uniformed personnel, mixing of males and females on wards, school for hospitalized teenagers, day care, and day hospital programs. Also explored were parental attitudes toward visiting the hospitalized adolescent, friendships their teenagers formed among patients and staff, ward activities, the hospital staff, and crises arising on the ward.

In the beginning of the study it had been assumed that there would be a high correlation between positive or negative attitudes of parents toward the hospital experience and adaptation of the hospitalized adolescents, but we were unable to find any significant correlations. The major factors involved in the evident neutrality of parents' feelings about their child's hospitalization and

Based on work by Betty Ann Glasser.

treatment were the preconceived ideas Bostonians knowledgeable about mental health had toward the MMHC.

Preconceived Attitudes

In middle-class families, definite status is associated with having a disturbed teenager admitted to the Harvard-staffed collegiate atmosphere of the MMHC. These patients considered it just as difficult for sick children to be admitted into this hospital, the principal psychiatric teaching facility for Harvard Medical School, as it is for healthy adolescents to be admitted to Harvard College, and would go to great lengths to use "pull." They would call upon their congressman, relatives and friends who are Harvard-connected. They also sent family members who may be "alumni" of the hospital to enlist the aid of hospital staff members.

For some parents the atmosphere of the MMHC creates the illusion that admission is equated with "success." Under these circumstances, parents are oblivious to any critical observations, at least during the early period of treatment. They tend to abdicate with relief all responsibility and leave the initiative to the hospital in whose preconceived omnipotence they invest their faith. Indeed, one of the major tasks of the social worker in casework is to re-engage parents as allies in the battle for their child's health.

In addition to preconceived attitudes of esteem and respect for the hospital, the parents brought along to the research interview their own built-in fears and phantasies about the underlying reason for the interview. Many felt guilty because their hospital bill was not paid, many hurried to the interview prepared to hear that their child was doing something intolerable that might jeopardize his hard-won place in the hospital. Many believed that patients were transferred "at the drop of a hat" when relatives became too bothersome and were worried about something they themselves might have done.

Initially, only a few parents were secure enough to feel relaxed. In almost all cases the first half of the interview time was devoted to reassurances that the purpose of the interview was not to discuss hospital bills or to break bad news and that nothing they said in the interests of research would be held against them or their hospitalized child. With the exception of two parents who remained unconvinced and insisted on being put on record as saying that "everything was perfect," parents were then able to sit back in their chairs, to enjoy the idea of being asked their views about the hospital experience, and to talk freely.

FEELINGS ABOUT HOSPITALIZING A CHILD

For most parents hospitalization was a traumatic experience, although almost all of them, as mentioned previously, experienced a feeling of relief at having the burden of the care and responsibility of the sick adolescent lifted from the shoulders of the family. Some mothers mentioned being involved in minor auto accidents while driving their child to the hospital; others said they had been unable to drive at all.

HOSPITAL ADMISSION

The hospital admission procedure, whereby family and patient are served coffee in a pleasant sitting room with a doctor, social worker and nurse present, was usually, by design, a pleasant one, and only when something went wrong—papers were not in order, the doctor could not be located, or a long, unexpected wait in the lobby ensued—was the initial impression of the hospital unfavorable.

Parents were apt to visit too often at first in response to pleas and demands of their children to be taken home; half of the adolescents had never been away from home for much more than a week's time. They also came in response to their own feelings of anxiety and helplessness, for it was hard for them to assess the legitimacy of their children's complaints. Common complaints were dislikes of roommates or of other patients, inability to get along with other patients, accusation of alcoholism, homosexuality, and sexual acting-out, fear of specific patients, inability to sleep, poor food, constant restrictions, and dissatisfaction with school setup. Although almost all of the adolescents suffered difficulties and adjustment problems during the first few months, parents reported active rebellion against hospitalization in only nine cases.

PROBLEMS DURING THE FIRST MONTHS

During the first months of hospitalization, parents worried about having adults of the opposite sex sleeping next door to their child's room. All whose children were not in the new wards were disappointed by the condition and appearance of the wards and resented having their children housed in such quarters. Other difficulties mentioned concerned their children's reaction to medication, frequent inability to reach the patient by telephone, and lack of structured activity. Most parents found the frequent traveling to and from their homes (the MMHC admits from all over Massachusetts) exhausting, and gradually were able to reduce their visits to weekly ones and to alternate visits between husband and wife.

ATTITUDES TOWARD HOSPITAL POLICIES

During the first months, the open-door policy proved to be a great source of concern to the parents whose children were constantly leaving the hospital without permission and then being put on restrictions so that they were not allowed to go home weekends or leave the hospital when their parents visited. The majority of parents, however, preferred the open door policy to locked wards and barred windows.

The whole subject of restrictions was a sore one for almost all parents of children not in the day hospital. There was more confusion, hard feelings and indignation generally in this area of hospital policy than in any other. Parents complained of never knowing whether their child would be able to come home for the weekend or not. They often felt that the restrictions were being unfairly placed on them when their children were not allowed to go home on holidays, weekends, and school vacations. "Spending Mother's Day visiting my son at MMHC is something I wouldn't wish on my worst enemy," one woman said bitterly. "The place was so dark, empty, deserted-looking. What a punishment for me! I went home and couldn't sleep all night."

Their attitude was more positive toward the idea of nurses and attendants wearing ordinary street clothes and toward patients and staff eating together. There were some feelings that the school as set up had little to offer, but most parents were extremely grateful for two classrooms and two public school teachers within the hospital.

Parents whose children were in the day hospital (5 of the 27 interviewed) seemed to be more satisfied with all hospital policies, staff, etc. than the others. Their satisfaction might have been a result of the fact that they did not experience feelings of guilt at having hospitalized their children or that they came to grips more quickly with their problems since they were responsible for caring for the patients more hours of the day than was the hospital.

VISITING

With few exceptions parents preferred to bear the burden of visiting their hospitalized children alone or with immediate family members such as older siblings or grandparents and other relatives living in the home. Sometimes visiting was a pleasant experience; patients would be listening to music, playing chess, cards, reading, so that the illusion was that of a day room in a country club or college dormitory. Some days the whole ward would be high; there would be crying, swearing, inappropriate laughing—not a pleasant sight for visitors. Then, too, parents never knew what to expect of their children. Many dreaded the visit not knowing whether they would be greeted with curses, shouts of "Get away from me!", or by a sullen and subdued greeting preceding a hostile silence or monosyllabic negative responses to any question. Often their children would hide from them or would suddenly demand to be taken out to eat or make other inappropriate requests. For example, one adolescent kept asking his parents for money for other patients. Parents universally voiced a wish for the comforting presence of someone on the wards during visiting hours to whom they could turn to for direction and guidance. The nurses and attendants were too busy or looked too preoccupied to be approached as they walked by. Many parents admitted spending their visiting time talking with other patients or with other parents.

ATTITUDES TOWARD ADOLESCENTS ON ADULT WARDS

When questioned about their attitudes toward having their child live on an adult ward, the majority of parents admitted not knowing what to answer. They apparently had given no thought as to the reason their child was not on a ward with peers of the same sex or in a special children's unit. Invariably their reply was, in essence, "If you people think it's good, who am I to say?" In fact, of the entire Cohort, only one parent complained that she did not want her son with disturbed old men. Furthermore, the social workers reported that none of the parents ever brought up the subject in casework except in relation to disapproval and anxiety about their children being on the same ward as "court cases." This does not actually relate to any feeling about adults being on the same ward with their children, since many of the "court cases" were adolescents themselves, but more to anxieties about "bad influences."

ATTITUDES TOWARD PEER RELATIONSHIPS

Parents had ambivalent feelings when some of the adolescents became fast friends with other hospitalized adolescents. They worried equally about their children associating with the wrong people—peers who could exert a bad influence on them or older "court cases"—or not associating with anybody at all. Although parents were impressed by the general high intelligence and calibre of the patient population, they expressed concern about how many of the patients on the wards were suicidal or used violent and foul language.

They were also concerned about the attachments their children formed to young attendants or student nurses and feared that their child would be doubly bereft when the student nurse or student attendant had to leave.

ATTITUDES TOWARD STAFF AND TREATMENT

Most of the parents found their social workers a source of support and comfort and had positive attitudes toward the doctors and ward personnel as well. A major attitude expressed about the ward personnel was that they were "nice," but kept their distance where relatives were concerned. Of the sixteen parents (largely mothers) who belonged to groups led by a staff psychiatrist, half found the group experience helpful and half did not. The common complaint of those who did not was that the doctor who led the group "would not answer questions."

Most parents expressed a wish that they be able to see their child's doctor more often; some had never been able to speak to him at all. Basically the wish was founded more on anxiety about what the doctors thought about them as parents and the desire to get the doctor on their side (many parents had the feeling that their child's therapist "was against them") than on an actual desire for more information. Much time was spent in casework discussing how and why Dr. So-and-so could walk right by a parent without so much as a nod of recognition. And in fact young residents often did shy away from greeting parents in the hospital lobby, hallways, and on the wards because they did not want to be asked to side with the parent in family quarrels.

Certainly in cases where the adolescents were on drugs, the parents would be justified in wanting to talk to the doctor when questions arose about side effects, dosages, or taking pills when home weekends. Likewise certain family issues arose in treatment pertaining to parents feeling that their child hated them, for example, or an adolescent feeling that his parents hated him, where, it seems family group sessions would indeed be indicated.

ATTITUDES TOWARD WARD CRISES

Almost all parents were aware of occasional crises on the wards such as attempts at suicide, deaths, inappropriate sexual activity, escapes, transfers to other state hospitals, and in fact worried excessively about the possibility of such occurrences. When the crises actually occurred, however, it was difficult for parents to talk about them. At the time of the two major crises reported in Chapter 4, social workers reported few direct references to these incidents in casework interviews with the parents of adolescent patients. In instances where the social worker initiated the discussion about the crisis and its effect upon the adolescents in general, usually the parent had known about the incident and was pathetically grateful for any crumb that could be offered in the way of assurance that their child might be immune from the contagion of the crises.

CONCLUSIONS

Positive or negative attitudes on the part of parents toward the hospital experience appeared to bear little or no relationship to their child's hospital course. They were generally pleased with hospital policies and thought new methods were being explored to benefit the patients. Yet parents did speak of being concerned about the wards their children were on, their roommates, their associates, their lack of activity, their exposure to foul language, alcoholism, overt sexual activity, and bizarre behavior. But they did little or nothing about these concerns since they were generally uncertain about being right or being worthy of venturing an opinion. Parental attitudes toward the hospital experience fit in with our picture of the character structure of these parents, of their feelings of inadequacy and inferiority as people in general and as parents in particular.

PART IV

Issues of Therapeutic Management

When the adolescent is a patient, control of impulsive behavior, especially in an environment as permissive as the wards of the MMHC, is an everpresent problem. "Setting limits" and "firm consistency" become key phrases in dealing with adolescents, and the management of these patients was an everpresent topic at morning report, in parents' groups, and in casework.

CHAPTER 8

Issues and Problems: The Adolescent and the Therapist

This chapter represents the views of the principal psychiatrists involved in this project concerning the issues and problems in the treatment of adolescents as they arose in our setting and as they are likely to arise in any similar setting.

ISSUES AND PROBLEMS:

Admission:

The first issue relates to the clinical characteristics of the adolescent study population admitted to the hospital. It is clear that they were on the whole severely ill. Since there was a limit on hospital beds available for adolescents, essentially those with severe behavior disturbance and no other place to go were hospitalized.

Based on work by Gertrude Rogers and Milton Greenblatt.

Some were acting out against the environment, attempting self-destruction, or had tormented their families to such a degree that they had often "reached the end of their rope." Another group of patients was so bizarre and frightening in their conduct that parents felt forced to ask for their separation from home. Our patients, then, were seriously ill clinically, usually in an acute state, often with a long history of difficulties preceding admission, and frequently acting out aggressively against the environment as a final episode leading to hospitalization.

Separation

Separation from the family was, of course, part of the fact of hospitalization. To the involved parties this could be, at one end of the spectrum, a serious trauma, and at the other end, a considerable relief. The overall clinical impression, however, was that in most instances it was a relief because parents and child had been caught up in a relational impasse so involving and pathological as to seriously impair the adolescent's development and maturation.

The separation was by no means easy. In fact it can be said that ambivalent elements were present in all instances, and that in some cases ambivalance was so extreme and active that both parents and child made many attempts to restore physical closeness, even when it seemed both unnecessary and unwise to professional observers. Many parents visited children too often and too long, abusing privileges that were already generous; they complained that their youngsters were unhappy, which indeed they often were; they listened to the adolescent's lamentations with total credulity, unable to see both sides; and they accused staff of lack of understanding of the patient's needs, tolerance, or down-right cruelty. When they were separated, the adolescent acted out in his ward while at home the parents created domestic "emergencies" requireing the patient's presence.

Therefore, one frequently encountered guilt, fear, depression, and feelings of abandonment in both the child and his parents. These were especially marked in the case of the youngster, and in various degrees, often seriously, these feelings interfered with his ability to utilize freely the therapeutic elements of the environment.

What separation often accomplished in a very positive sense, however, was to give the adolescent a new opportunity to utilize his interests and energies—an opportunity to make relationships with a wide variety of helpful persons, to absorb the therapeutic culture with its new values and rich activities. Distance from home and parents also allowed old sores to heal. It is true that battles so heatedly fought in the family setting were delayed in their final solution; but, as a matter of fact as well as of theory, in the opinion of most observers their ultimate working through was generally aided by the growth of the adolescent during his period of hospitalization.

Continuity of Staff

Continuity of staff, highly desirable in any therapeutic environment, was in this case a critical factor. In view of the large staff-patient ratio, the urban situation of the hospital, and its essential teaching responsibilities, the turnover was considerable. For each ward of twenty-eight patients including four adolescents, there might be a complete changeover of the five or six residents at the end of each year, not to mention nursing and attendant staff, social workers, and others. At the end of the year, by the time the resident became comfortable with the adolescent, his training program often mandated a move to another ward. From the standpoint of the treatment needs of many patients, it might have been desirable to have fewer residents and more long-term staff persons, but the large training commitment precluded such solution. The above stresses are perhaps inevitably related to the multiple goals of a teaching institution.

Ratio of Adolescents to Adults

Anyone using a plan similar to ours will have to decide what ratio of adolescents to adults is best when the two are intermingled for treatment purposes. We reasoned that a predominance of adults would mean that adolescents would feel strongly the restraining influence of adult behavior, values, and conditioning; on the other hand, several adolescents together on such a ward would be able to share problems, give each other support, and enjoy socio-recreational activities together. Thus we arbitrarily chose a ratio of four adolescents to twenty-four or twenty-six adults—making a total average ward population of twenty-eight to thirty patients. Whether this *is* the optimum ratio remains for experience or research to determine. We did not experiment systematically with varying ratios, although we would strongly recommend that it be done. It seems obvious, however, that a *single* adolescent on an adult ward would pose special problems, including loneliness, lack of feeling of belonging, and therapeutic opportunity to be with peers; however, a large number of adolescents on an adult ward would at some point threaten the balance between order and impulse that we tried to establish. All that we can say is that our judgment concerning ratio of adolescents/adults turned out to be a reasonable one, in terms of a workable therapeutic organization under the particular conditions that prevailed.

Identification between Young People

On these wards, many of the staff and even "adult" patients were young. The fact that adolescents were being treated by young people raised real problems. On the one hand, the young people tended to identify readily with each other, perhaps often to overidentify, with the risk of unwise involvement in emotional affairs; on the other hand, there was the risk of staff being frightened or outraged by the adolescents' unstable and bizarre behavior. The student nurse, the youthful volunteer, and the young resident often found it difficult, therefore, to take the ups and downs of the adolescent's life. Long experience was required to maintain one's equanimity in relation to shocking sexual fantasies, primitive rage, or rebellion. Sometimes behavior was epidemic; window-breaking and wrist-nicking, for example, were frequently contagious in the intensive ward milieu where unstable adolescents were able to reinforce one another's behavior.

To compensate for problems of overidentification and even lack of experience in such a ward was the fact that the adolescents possessed real feelings of sympathy for each other. Many of these youngsters were isolates on the outside; it was a great relief for them to know that others were dealing with similar problems and were suffering in similar ways.

Competition for Patients

To some extent, the adolescents were in a favored position; identification with them was strong, especially on the part of young nurses and residents, and therapeutic personnel were eager to work with them since there was always a relative "shortage" of adolescent patients. The adolescents at time used this situation in the service of their neurotic manipulations. Sometimes student nurses showered them with gifts or favors, or residents asked for exclusive therapeutic rights, arguing that the multiple-therapist situation was hard to control and that they were not equipped to assume leadership of a heterogeneous therapeutic team.

Student nurses were known to form closed diadic relationships with the adolescents, sharing together a feeling of "two against the world" or "only we understand each other." There was often evidence that adolescents were reacting to such secret relationships rather than to other relationships that were thought to be under control.

Control and Permissiveness

The application of controls was more of an issue in the treatment of the adolescent than of the adult; limits on the former's behavior were very frequently required. This was, of course, a result of their greater aggressiveness and their need to test the environment. Controls had to be planned carefully so that the whole staff could cooperate effectively, otherwise the manipulating patient would sense a break in the front of understanding and quickly take advantage of the situation. The main behavioral manifestations for which controls had to be applied were aggressiveness, destructiveness, belligerency, extravagant emotional displays such as temper tantrums, shrieking and yelling, sexual acting-out, going off limits before privileges were earned, and serious infraction of schedules concerning therapy hours and group activities. Generally, verbal request or admonitions were sufficient; however, in a few instances we had to exercise physical controls, although never until the problem was thoroughly discussed and we were convinced that this was the only method. The reasons for controls were carefully explained to the patient both by ward chief and nursing staff and then taken up in therapeutic sessions by psychiatrist or group therapist.

Some difficulties in exercising controls stemmed from the high staff turnover which increased the problem of transmission of information and/or attitudes from one person or group to the next. There was also the problem posed by the residues of adolescent rebellion in staff so that only by trial and error did one learn how tension was initiated and how to deal with it.

In some cases the problem of applying controls was not easily worked out, especially when staff opinion was divided as to merits and methodology regarding the individual case and clinical sessions with staff were not successful in reaching a consistent understanding. Not infrequently there was an interesting fluctuation between too much permissiveness for the given patient followed by compensatory reactions to the consequences of overpermissiveness. This, needless to say, made things unpredictable and uncomfortable for both patients and staff.

A further complication was that a few patients were subjected to severe controls, some to mild controls, while a great many were treated very permissively, all in the same environment. Practicing a broad range of attitudes toward different patients sometimes proved to be confusing. A final problem was that the overall atmosphere of the ward was generally on the permissive side so that enforcement of controls in individual cases was often difficult to carry out.

Educational Therapy

In this particular setting there were two full time teachers appointed by the Boston school system and two classes running each day, corresponding to a community school. Although there was no participation by the hospital in the choice of teachers, we felt that selection was made by the city authorities with care and consideration. Once the teachers were chosen an effort was made to develop them as responsible allies in therapy. It was planned that "teacher development" include frequent meetings between members of the treatment staff and the teachers to obtain information, to share problems, and to provide interpretation about the patient's behavior. In practice, however, meetings were few and far between because of conflicts in time. It was found necessary to assign an attendant as liason between the staff and the school, available to the teachers during school hours to escort problematic adolescents back to their wards.

Some of the most disturbed children responded well to the structure of the school program. This may be surprising, to some but not to those who are familiar with child and adolescent mental problems. In the classroom some of the adolescents showed impressive ability and areas of strength not suspected before.

One of the values of the school is to make it possible for the adolescent to sit with others in a structured group situation in close contact. The structured situation is a reminder of their earliest school days; it is a revival of older conditioning in a corrective atmosphere. The classroom situation also affords the adolescent the opportunity to sublimate through intellectualization, to learn something useful and practical, and to develop deepening relationships with other members of a growing, changing group.

THE ADOLESCENT AND THE THERAPIST

It was generally assumed that the adolescent was an unfolding, developing personality and that anything that impinged on him at this critical stage might make a difference in terms of his growth. It was also assumed that growth could be facilitated or catalyzed by a wide array of possible interventions, including psychotherapy, group therapy, social activities, work, rehabilitation, occupational therapy, drugs, school, and adventures and experiments in community living in the form of going out into the city or town and joining with the general public.

The assumption of the staff was that psychotherapy with adolescents was more than simply talking to patients and trying to gain insight. It was far more important to be "in touch" with the adolescent and know what was going on within him, to have some sense and appreciation of his struggles, and to be aware of his attempts to establish control. "I see the therapist as catalyzing growth in this special sense and intervening where the adolescent is not able to make use of available resources," said one of our senior psychiatrists. Staff were cautioned to be wise about avoiding "digging" or standard uncovering techniques that are so often utilized in work with adult neurotics. Since therapy was to a large extent in the hands of untrained resident psychiatrists, it was stressed repeatedly that the adolescent often has a problem of too little rather than too much repression and is in danger of being overwhelmed by opening his Pandora's Box. We did not suggest that psychotherapy should be superficial but that a wise balance should be made between uncovering explosive material and helping the adolescent maintain his personality structure.

Patient Therapist Relationship*

Observation about the adaptive patterns within therapy indicates that there is a wide range of ways in which therapist and adolescent patient try to reach each other in order to communicate. Although to a greater or lesser extent difficulties and disruptions beset each relationship, we were repeatedly struck by the phenomenon of therapist and patient trying over and over again to make themselves understood to the other, of giving each other many a "second" chance at times of rebuffs and misunderstanding. Thus, once the initial contact has been established, both therapist and patient are obviously motivated to relate to each other, albeit at times through highly defensive, distorted, or primitive means. This phenomenon in itself seems important in view of the particular complications added to the therapy relationship by the fact that the patient is an adolescent and the therapist is an adult.

We might assume that any hospitalized patient has found himself too vulnerable to psychic pain or tension to have been able to face or adequately deal with it and has taken flight from such tension at the expense of contact with reality, For the adolescent this flight is also at the expense of his further development or growth toward adulthood at that point. Therapy, both in the classical sense and with the use of the environmental adjuncts, aims to strengthen the tension-bearing capacities of the adolescent's ego sufficiently so that he can continue his development through the progressive forces in his personality. For the adolescent, with the developmental tasks of establishing a separate identity and resolving his infantile ties, an intense relationship with an adult can be as dangerous as is it potentially supportive. The need to liberate himself from his own regressive wishes is often expressed as a revolution against the adults he still needs. Yet if the adult fails to provide him with firm controls, the disturbed adolescent experiences this as a loss of protection from the impulses which are frightening to him, and panics, with disastrous results. Thus the adolescent, convinced that he has been controlled for the benefit of others, must come to believe that

---

* Based on interviews by Lora Heims Tessman with resident therapists.

the therapist (even, or especially, when he sets limits) is on his side and cares. The therapist of the disturbed adolescent frequently must straddle the psychic fence of offering himself freely as a new identification figure and a protective ally of the ego while avoiding the over-stimulation of those impulses and regressive ties against which the adolescent is attempting to protect himself. We are well aware that even for unusually flexible and sensitive therapists who like adolescents and find them gratifying to work with, the adolescent patient is at times most taxing and evokes defense and self-protective maneuvers on the part of the therapist.

Analysis of our observations suggests that there are dynamic changes during therapy in the therapist's view of his patient. This occurs not only in regard to such aspects as prognosis but also in regard to relatively enduring aspects of the personality which the therapist may or may not value such as "intelligence." Thus, for example, during a period when psychotherapy was progressing well, one therapist commented on how gratifying this patient was to work with because he was so bright and articulate and would probably go on to college without trouble after hospitalization. About two months later, after the patient had broken four appointments in a row and acted as though he preferred the ward attendant to the therapist, the therapist commented that this patient was so much less interesting than his other, new adolescent patient because the former was more limited in intelligence and would probably never be "college material." Further associations indicated that this therapist was trying to convey that this patient was no longer smart enough to "know a good thing when he saw one"—namely the therapist.

Although there are individual differences, there are certain aspects of the patient's symptomatology and pathological behavior that are relatively easily tolerated by the therapist and are not a major threat to his self-esteem. Among these are regressive, infantile behavior (e.g., needing to be fed); demandingness directed toward the therapist (asking for more therapy time); and a bizarre but rich fantasy life. There are major differences in the ways in which the therapist reacted to bizarre material or primary process communications. These vary from the therapist who prided herself on how quickly she learned what she called "schizophrenese" in order to communicate with the patient in her terms to the therapist who each day patiently and silently waited until the patient finished with the bizarre verbalizations and then asked how she felt about her parents. One therapist showed anxiety when the patient wove him glibly into pregnancy fantasies which she tried to publicize on the ward. However, no therapist manifested a real withdrawal or aggression toward the patient in relation to the bizarre fantasy life.

In contrast, marked negative countertransference was noticeable in regard to the following behavior on the part of the patient:

(1) When the patient directly rejects what the therapist had to offer. This could frequently be seen after the patient had broken appointments, refused to stay in the therapy room with the therapist, refused to talk, or emotionally withdrew from the therapist for long periods of time.

(2) When the therapist feels manipulated by the patient. The therapist, and the hospital, placed a strong value on the therapist's being in command of the therapeutic interaction. The therapist was often told, concerning a wide variety of behavior by his patient ranging from asking for extra privileges to making suicidal attempts late at night, that "he is just trying to control you." The implication to the therapist seemed to be that he was being made a fool of by his patient and therefore must put a stop to the misbehavior immediately. This resulted at times in a retaliatory countertransference reaction in which the therapist quickly made clear to the patient that it was he, the therapist, who was in control. Although in many cases the result was a therapeutically correct one, in others the "manipulative" behavior was a healthier pattern than the patient's previous withdrawal, and the rejection with which it was met was unfortunate.

Within the complex vicissitudes of the therapist's relationship to his patients, we discerned a number of specific devices used by the therapist in an attempt to establish a close relationship with his patient and yet maintain a therapeutic distance and avoid in overidentification with the patient. Some examples were:

(1) Intellectualization about the patient, used in the interests of withdrawal by the therapist. This device was most often employed when the theoretical discussion about the patient served primarily to emphasize how different the patient was from the therapist.

(2) Projection of negative countertransference onto other staff members. This occurred when the therapist described how the rest of the staff rejected the patient for his obnoxious behavior, but he, the therapist, was not annoyed. Although this mechanism may have helped solidify the relationship initially, it was either apt to break down when the patient's behavior continued and the therapist admitted his own anger, or the patient and the therapist became a highly mutually identified pair, unified in steeling themselves against the depriving world.

(3) Negation of aspects of the personality of the patient which would be threatening to the therapist. Although this mechanism also served to maintain positive countertransference and identification with the patient for a time, the difficulty seemed to be that, as long as the need to deny an aspect of the patient's personality was in effect, the patient's needs and problems in this area could not be dealt with. Thus, for example, one therapist described her adolescent girl patient as "just a likeable little girl" and could not understand why others considered her sexually seductive. The therapist did not think of her as a "bad girl." When this girl increased her sexualized behavior until the therapist saw this too, there was a serious disruption of the therapeutic relationship, and the therapist felt that patient's prognosis was suddenly very poor.

Vicissitudes of Therapy with Adolescents

The psychiatric residents on the whole were deeply interested in their task and highly identified with the patients. Their supervision was supplied by experienced child psychiatrists, usually one hour a week for each adolescent in individual therapy.

The first problem that the resident usually faced was that the clinical condition of the adolescent was more fluid that that of the adult, there were more ups and downs and the therapeutic relationship was more unstable. Because of the intense identification on the part of many of the therapists with the patient, the first defeat was often a serious narcissistic blow. This was much truer in work with adolescents than with adult patients, partly, of course, because the residents had less experience with the former. Because of the personal meaning of the defeat the resident was often not as supportive to the patient as he could have been and was too ready to give up.

A second problem was that the adolescent had difficulty bringing charged psychological material to his resident; thus the case was often regarded as disappointing, and there was less that the resident could report to his supervisor. This was usually interpreted to the resident as a familiar phase in the development of a relationship with an adolescent and not a reflection upon his abilities as a psychotherapist.

Another problem had to do with the interpretation of the transference. With fairly well-integrated adults, positive and negative transference could often be interpreted freely, but the resident has had to be highly selective about this in the case of the adolescent. Analysis of negative transference seemed often to yield good results, the adolescent responding with less hostile behavior. Analysis of the positive transference, however, was often disappointing, turning the adolescent away from his therapist. Since positive ties were often very tenuous and unstable, premature analysis of these ties frequently weakened them. There was also the component that the adolescent is frightened to get too close to anyone, especially a learned authority figure such as the resident appears to be.

In the supervision of residents, it frequently became necessary to recommend more freedom and license in their work to help the patient with his discovery of values and cultural patterns that are normally sanctioned. Since the adolescent is in a very active phase of trial and test, he sometimes profits greatly by simple explanations of why people behave the way they do in adult life. Residents were taught that the instructional, educative part of the relationship, with great emphasis on ego-building and support was generally to be emphasized more with an adolescent than it would be with an adult.

Corollary to the above was the importance of the therapist not appearing as a collaborator or participant when the adolescent acted out. If the adolescent considered him a collaborator, he was devalued as a therapist, and the adolescent's antisocial behavior was consequently reinforced.

Inexperienced psychotherapists had a tendency to set unrealistic goals for their adolescent patients. It is better in the case of adolescents to keep an open-ended view of progress, i.e., to set flexible goals and to consider therapy as of several years' duration with progressive revision over time. When this was not done the adolescent felt that too much was expected of him, and a sense of desperation cast its shadow upon the relationship.

Important difficulties occurred in relation to the fact that residents did not stay on forever; frequently the adolescent had to be transferred from one resident to another. This was often a highly traumatic period, and the July 1 turnover was accompanied by acting-out behavior on the part of the adolescents. They ran away, made suicidal gestures, became belligerent or withdrawn. A key technique in avoiding such developments was to help the resident *not* to become too central a figure in the patient's life. He was asked to encourage the patient to distribute his energies and emotional commitments widely so that when the therapist had to retreat the patient would be left with sufficient props to weather the storm. Thus, his relationship to nurses, attendants, adult patients, and other adolescents was to be facilitated in this environment. It was obvious that the resident's narcissism often required special attention from his supervisors in this area.

The resident was taught that preparation of the patient for the reality of the resident's leaving was to be part of the initial contract in therapy, and discussion of feelings with respect to this eventuality could occur whenever the patient needed it. It was also important that if staff members were scheduled to leave the institution they did not discuss this event with others before they communicated it to the patient.

One of the most dramatic problems in therapy with adolescents, especially in a setting with a large staff turnover and numerous opportunities to communicate tension to others, was the tendency for adolescents to express themselves by dramatic outrageous behavior. Minor epidemics of slashing, swallowing pins or glass, etc. did occur. The slashings occurred mainly in severely emotionally deprived girls who had problems of a hostile dependent relationship with their mothers and probably considerable latent homosexuality, and who now were being cared for by female staff. This phenomenon was sometimes very difficult to predict. The staff anxieties about episodes were likely to intensify the epidemics. On such occasions one supported strongly the ward staff, especially the resident psychotherapist. With reduction of tension all around and less fear concerning risk of death, these phenomena became less frequent and troublesome.

There were of course numerous other issues and problems in the course of hospitalization, as there would be with any group of patients in any hospital, which could be discussed at great length. We have chosen to discuss in this chapter only the issues that appeared to apply specifically to the adolescent population of the MMHC: specifically problems connected with admission to the hospital and separation from the family; problems of management in terms of type of staff, ratio of adolescents to adult patients, and the general problem of control versus permissiveness; and especially a whole series of problems arising in the interaction of the adolescent patient and the resident psychiatrist.

CHAPTER 9

Problems Parents Brought to Casework

At the MMHC it has long been a policy that casework should be available for the immediate family of patients and that the main focus of social work in the hospital be on the treatment of the family. It has been traditional for the social workers to assess, through an interview or series of intake interviews with the relatives of patients, the social situation at admission and then to offer casework contact with the relatives through one of the following four approaches: (1) short-term supportive, (2) long-term supportive, (3) long-term self-awareness, and (4) short telephone contacts with family in moments of crisis.

It is useful to image a spectrum running from: "What has he/she done?" to "What have I done?" There is a mixture of these aspects in every case. When more of the former is present, the casework will tend to be just supportive, helping the family live through a difficult situation; when more of the latter is present, the casework can more readily move toward focusing on awareness if not of self, then of the relationship between the patient and the family.

The Adolescent Unit considered it imperative that a strong effort be made to keep patients of adolescents in treatment and in some cases made this a condition of the adolescent's hospitalization.

To find out what the caseworker did to help the families of these adolescents with their problems, we perused the case records of the Cohort and examined the content of casework contacts and the function of the caseworker. What were the dominant themes which parents brought into casework and to what extent and in what context did the problem of controlling and managing the adolescent come up in casework? We were also interested in the extent of casework contact with these families in a time sequence, such as pre-hospitalization, at intake, during hospitalization, and after discharge, as well as the duration of contact.

Based on work by Shelley Erhlich and Libby Herrera

Data from casework records for a two-year period on adolescents in the Cohort were collected on a precoded schedule. Of the fifty-five patients under study, in one case the parents or relatives were not seen at all, fourteen were seen for intake interviews only, and eighteen had contact with a social worker less than eight months. Only twenty-two parents or relatives (40 per cent) had a long-term treatment relationship with a social worker.

In all but a small percentage of instances, it was the mother who was seen regularly. Although it was recognized that both parents were important to the patient and responsible for taking part in treatment, only a few fathers were willing to take time off from their working day to talk with the social worker, and only a few social workers were willing either to insist that they do or to make evening or weekend appointments on a regular basis.

Although it was considered important for both parents to participate in group therapy, in only seven cases were both involved in such a group. In seven other cases, just the mother attended the group. In all fourteen of these cases, the parents were also being seen both together and separately by individual caseworkers, and contact was quite consistent and regular, generally on a long-term basis. Although this appears to be an unusually involved group of parents, achievement of social work goals was not obviously greater in this group than it was within the total Cohort, probably because of the severe degree of illness in this particular group of parents which made casework goals difficult to attain in one or two years, if ever.

Goals of casework with parents of the thirty-seven patients about whom information is available from the records are listed below. As could be expected, giving support of one type or another evolved as the predominant role of the caseworker.

Goals	*No. of Cases Cited*
Support	
a) give to mother so mother can give to child	26
b) help handle alleviate guilt	
c) help parent improve self-image	
d) help parent ventilate feelings (anger) toward patient	

Help parent gain insight into own relationship with patient	13
Help parents set limits or controls for patient	11
Help parent accept need for hospitalization and interpret illness	9
Information gathering	9
Help parent see patient realistically as an individual and understand his needs and anxieties	7
Help parent plan for post hospitalization	7
Establish relationship with hostile parents	5
Interpretation of hospital management, policy, program, and limits	5
Help with marital relationship	4

Casework services, through setting up a therapeutic process for the parents, provided the richest source of material on family relationships. Of the fifty-five families in the Cohort, thirty-seven complete casework recordings exist. These records revealed many signs of the disorder and disequilibrium that dominate the families of these disturbed adolescents.

The parents brought into casework problems that could well be categorized as a "dilemma of parental self-identity.:[4] unresolved feelings of dissatisfaction and inadequacy, chronic marital discord, conflictual relationships with the extended family, and confusion over the management of adolescent behavior.

DESCRIPTION OF THE PARENTS

A common denominator in the lives of these parents was their overwhelming feelings of guilt and anxiety over the mental illness of their adolescent children. The quality of these feelings permeated much of the other content found in the casework records.

The description of this group of mothers (and the same procedure was followed for the fathers) was made in terms of the mothers' directly expressed or implied feelings of adequacy or in-

---

[4] Literland, T. and Smith, I.: The dilemma of self-identity in parents of psychotic children. *Social Work Practice,* New York and London Columbia University Press, 1962.

adequacy, satisfaction or dissatisfaction—as wife, mother, daughter and as a person.

Although there were many themes and minor variations, our study of these mothers of thirty-seven hospitalized adolescents produced one predominating impression. What emerged was the picture of a group of mothers who were mostly chronically dissatisfied with themselves, with their families of origin, and with their current families. The largest group of these mothers expressed moderate to severe dissatisfaction in all these spheres. In describing these feelings, some mothers tended to focus the material on their own disturbed relationships with their mothers. Others focused on the marital situation, and still others on their relationship to their children or more specifically to the patient. In many instances the mother's feelings of frustration and inadequacy colored most of the casework content. A small group of mothers were considered to be borderline psychotic or to show marked neurotic symptoms.

Our attempt to gain a picture of the fathers posed a special problem not encountered with the mothers. Material on the father was most often given to the caseworker by the mother, the more frequent client. It was also gained infrequently from sporadic casework contact with the father. Many of the fathers remained obscure to the caseworker: we did not know their feelings about themselves as husband, father, son, or person. This obscurity may have been suggestive of limitations in our interest or services to the father, or it may have been symptomatic of the father's relationship with the mother and the total family.

What information we have about the fathers suggested one predominant category: the passive-dependent type. These fathers seemed to abnegate their authority in the family. It was the wives who took the major responsibility for decisions and for rearing of the children. The fathers seemed to relate passively to their disturbed adolescent; they often remained in the shadowy background, leaving the mother alone to handle the complicated and painful experience of hospitalizing the adolescent. In addition, some were described by the workers as severely disturbed or borderline; about one-third were known to have been hospitalized for alcoholism or other mental illness.

The material on family separation and losses indicated that many of the adolescents had to deal at one time or another with the physical loss of their fathers from the home. The above description of the fathers strongly suggests that many of these adolescents likewise had to cope with an inadequate emotional relationship with a less than adequate father.

MARITAL RELATIONSHIPS

A crucial factor in the life of the family is the nature of the marital relationship. A problem which is continually brought to casework treatment by these parents was that of severe marital conflict. In the majority of these families the onset of marital conflict occurred prior to the adolescent's illness, antedating the beginning of adolescence in many of the children, often beginning as far back as the early childhood of the now troubled adolescent. The vicissitudes of the adolescent children seem to exacerbate the unresolved problems of the individual parent and of the marital relationship. The discord between the parents was evidenced frequently in conflict over the rearing of the children. The expression of marital maladjustment among these families ranged from silent hostility between the parents to a state of open and violent warfare.

It has been suggested in a study done by the Harvard University School of Public Health of one hundred and sixteen mothers of normal adolescents that the most important factor in sustaining the mother during the strains and stresses of her child's adolescence is a secure, sustaining relationship with her husband.[5] The mothers in our study did not have close, supportive relationships with their husband and brought to casework their feelings of vulnerability in dealing with the problems of their disturbed teenager.

MANAGEMENT AND CONTROL OF THE ADOLESCENT

In the casework setting the predominant concern of all of the parents was how to manage the behavioral problems of the adolescent. In seeking help with how to cope with the adolescent's behavior during hospital visits and more urgently during the patient's home visits, the parents gave a rich description of the overt areas of conflict between the adolescents and themselves. Underlying some of the difficulty in managing the adolescent was the

---

[5] Butler R.; Mother's attitudes toward the social development of their adolescents: Part II. *Social Casework,* June, 1956.

parents' own uncertainty as to the boundary between normal adolescent rebelliousness and psychiatric symptoms. The parents felt at a loss to understand the transitory, fluctuating moods of the adolescent. This sense of confusion was further compounded by the parents' unfamiliarity both with the psychiatric disorders and with the psychotherapeutic approach of the hospital to these problems.

Inability to set reasonable limits and controls on the adolescent characterized much of the parental approach. In most instances the parents' vacillation in setting limits predates hospitalization. This problem was further intensified by the mobilization of guilt feelings attendant on hospitalizing the adolescent. The overt conflicts between the adolescent and his parents extended into three spheres: the adolescent's personal behavior, his interpersonal relationships within the family, and his social behavior. The latter two categories appeared in the casework records with greater intensity and frequency.

Parents' dissatisfaction with how the adolescent cares for his physical self was expressed in the areas of food consumption and physical grooming. A few parents expressed their relationship with the adolescent primarily in involvement over the consumption of food. Another small group of parents complained that the adolescent was slovenly in appearance, which was intolerable. Relatively few parents, however, focussed on these potential areas of conflict; most were concerned about the familial and social relationships of the adolescent.

FAMILY INTERRELATIONSHIPS

Within the immediate family the areas of conflict centered on temper tantrums, unrealistic demand of attention and goods, stubbornness, willful disobedience, insolence, and disrespect. It is in trying to manage these behavioral problems that the parent most frequently seeks and utilizes casework help. Regardless of the etiology of these problems, the parents were confronted with how best to cope with this disruptive and unacceptable behavior. From this point of view, these problems were linked with the issue of how the parents helped the adolescent achieve appropriate control over his behavior.

Descriptive material on the siblings of these disturbed adolescents appeared in only about two-thirds of the thirty-five records studied.

These families can be divided into two groups of almost equal size. In the first group the parents were having moderate to severe difficulties with the siblings of the hospitalized adolescent. In the second group the parents described themselves as having a satisfying, minimally conflictual relationship with the siblings. We are dealing here, not with a diagnostic evaluation of siblings but with the parents' own perception and feelings about the sibling and their relationship to him. In some of these families there was a chronically hostile relationship between the hospitalized adolescent and his siblings. The parents were concerned about the effects of the adolescent's hospitalization on the other children in the family. They were also troubled about how to control the often aggressive, hostile behavior of the patient to his sibling during home visits or how much to expect the sibling to include the withdrawn patient into his own more normal social life.

In many families, a grandparent, usually the maternal grandmother, had a significant enough role in the family's life to have influenced the patient's childhood. In some cases the grandparent shared a common household with the family for several years. Other grandparents acted as mother substitutes, usually during the patient's infancy. Frequently both types of contact existed within the same family. For some families the relationship with the dominant grandparents continued until the patient was hospitalized. For others, in which the grandparents is now deceased, the relationship was an important part of the past history of the patient and his family and was frequently brought up in connection with assigning guilt for the adolescent's illness.

SOCIAL ADJUSTMENT

The social development of the adolescent was an important and complicated concern for parents. School adjustment and peer relationships encompass a large segment of social life. Disruption in school attendance or performance during hospitalization often became a focus for the parent's anxieties over the adolescent's future. The parent, beset by doubts as to what school achievement to expect from his troubled teenager, looked to the case worker for clarification.

Problems arising from peer and sexual relationships were mentioned very often. Many of the anxieties related in a distorted manner to these normal areas of parental concern: the parents were fearful the adolescent would become delinquent, that he would become sexually promiscuous, that he would prefer adult to peer relationships. Sometimes these fears stemmed from the patient's behavior or his symptomatology, and sometimes from the parent's own unresolved problems. In either case, the parent was faced with the task of understanding the adolescent's social needs and helping him to achieve them appropriately.

Conclusions

The content of casework with the families of thirty-seven hospitalized adolescents indicated that we were dealing with parents who themselves were moderately or severely disturbed. The mothers particularly described themselves as feeling most inadequate and dissatisfied in all their significant relationships. These chronic feelings were intensified by a mobilization of their own unresolved adolescent conflicts. The fathers appeared to take a subordinate position in family management and decision making. To these troubled waters were added not only the normal turbulence of adolescent children but the additional upheaval of a disturbed teenager requiring psychiatric intervention.

Although many of the problems these parents brought into casework are characteristic of disturbed parent-child relationships, they take on a quality particular to the needs of adolescence. The parent's own legitimate confusion between adolescent turmoil and psychiatric disorders colors much of his perception. The issue of management and control of behavior, a concern for all parents of adolescents, assumed enormous proportions for these parents.

CHAPTER 10

A Parent Therapy Group

Group psychotherapy with parents of hospitalized adolescents was organized with two purposes in mind: to evaluate such a group as a therapeutic tool within this setting and as a means of increasing our understanding of adolescent patients and their families. The group, originally composed of four couples, met once a week and continued for a year and a half.

In contrast to the work of Bowen[6] and Ackerman,[7] who structured the group around major family members including the "patient," this group included only the mother and father and any other significant members of the family. In addition, its focus was primarily therapeutic, with the leader taking an active role in the investigation of the difficulties of the members. This differed from the group experience with parents of hospitalized adolescents reported by Grinspoon, Courtney and Bergen.[8] In their work the leader functioned primarily as an observer who encouraged discussion of the children.

The criteria established in the selection of members were: (1) the adolescent was in the hospital at the time the group was started and (2) mother and father were living together and not participating in any other group. The latter criterion had to be modified when only two of the four couples who fulfilled the requirements agreed to join. The next two couples contacted either had one or both members in other groups. Mrs. Olan belonged to a mother's group and the Rifkins were members of a group that included all family mem-

---

By Gerald Adler

[6] Bowen, M.: In Jackson, D. D. (Ed.): *Etiology of Schizophrenia.* New York, Basic Books, 1960 p. 346.

[7] Ackerman, N. W.: A study in family diagnosis. *Am J. Orthopsychiatry,* 26:66, 1965.

[8] Grinspoon, L. Courtney, M. A., and Bergen, H. M.: The usefulness of a structured parents group in rehabilitation, In Greenblatt, M., et al. (Eds.): *Mental Patients in Transition* Springfield, Ill. Charles C Thomas, 1961, p. 229.

bers of patients entering one of the hospital services. The eight members of the group were interviewed individually or as a couple before the first meeting.

Since the chief criterion for entry into the group was the presence of a hospitalized adolescent in the family, the membership of course included people of different character structure and levels of functioning. It was assumed that the unifying force of such a heterogeneous group would be the common concern over the problem of a hospitalized child. The children all manifested seriously impaired ego-functioning at the time the group started. Two were unquestionably schizophrenic, one was a severe obsessive compulsive with a probable schizophrenic process not too far beneath the surface, and one presented impulse-control problems, although several observers felt that she was psychotic.

Description of the Members

The Olans were a middle-class Jewish couple.* Mr. Olan was in his mid-forties and worked as an engineer. Mrs. Olan was five years younger and, in contrast to her controlled, carefully organized and articulate husband, responded with much more overt emotion in her relationships with people. She approached people readily, but withdrew into a pouting anger when she felt rebuked. Linda, the hospitalized patient, was sixteen and had two younger sisters whom the Olans described as normal. Linda had entered the Massachusetts Mental Health Center one and a half years prior to the first group meeting, with a diagnosis of acute schizophrenic reaction.

The Rifkins were the oldest couple in the group. They were of Jewish background and both in their mid to late fifties. Their only child, Ernest, aged fifteen, had been born after they had been married a considerable time. Both before and after Ernest's birth, the Rifkins' marital life was characterized by constant strife and repeated separations. Mrs. Rifkin was obese, tended to be gossipy, and quickly became friendly with all the hospital personnel. Mr. Rifkin was articulate and argumentative, and extremely sensitive to any remark which remotely threatened his autonomy. Ernest was admitted to the Massachusetts Mental Health Center eight months

---

* The Olans were the parents of Linda, the schizophrenic girl described in our second case study.

before the first group meeting—agitated, frightened, hallucinating, and delusional.

The Halls were of Protestant, New England background. Mr. Hall, in his early fifties, was tall, clean-cut, and tweedy. He remained aloof from people and tended to relate in a paternalistic and condescending manner. Mrs. Hall, several years younger than her husband, was graying and tired looking. She dressed neatly and spoke softly and clearly. She seemed overwhelmed by her daughter's hospitalization but, like her husband, tended to see the brighter side of all difficulties. One month before the group began, Sandy, aged seventeen, had been admitted because of increasing obsessional thinking and compulsions which did not permit her to function adequately in school or at home. Her two younger brothers were considered normal by the family.

The Davidoffs presented the most stormy emotional history of the four couples. Mr. Davidoff's difficulties began more than thirty years before, and in the seven years before the group started, he had been admitted repeatedly to mental hospitals. He had been diagnosed as a manic-depressive and during his over-active periods had passed bad checks and drunk excessively. His admissions, however, were precipitated by severe depressions accompanied by suicidal thoughts. At the time he joined the group, he tended to be silent and withdrawn, but when he spoke his hoarse voice was loud and insistent. His obesity, short stature, and his perioral grimacing gave him a somewhat grotesque, ape-like appearance. Born in Russia of lower-class Jewish parents, he came to the United States when very young and worked at a variety of jobs since then. Mrs. Davidoff was native-born and worked as a secretary both before and after the marriage. She was short, somewhat overweight, and dyed her hair red. Mrs. Davidoff felt that the other group members came from wealthier and more sophisticated backgrounds, and she tried hard to appear composed and refined. She tended to support everyone except her husband in a conventional platitudinous way. Initially, her prime concern about joining the group was that her husband's mental illness would become known but she felt, "I have two sick ones and can use help in dealing with them." Naomi, the hospitalized patient, was sixteen and was considered by her parents to be very different from her twenty-year-old sister who was attending college. Naomi entered the hospital one month before the group began because the Davidoffs could not control her late hours or absences from school.

TRENDS AND DEVELOPMENTS OF THE GROUP

The contract presented to the four couples was broadly stated: to give the members the opportunity to discuss their difficulties with their children, as well as any personal problems. The research purpose of the meetings was also mentioned. The group met in the early evening once a week for fifty minutes. In addition to the leader, a social worker was always present as a non-participating recorder.

The evolution of the group was consistent with the basic observations in the literature about group psychotherapy.[9] Hence the focus of this chapter will be confined to the unique aspects of the interaction of this group, and will omit many of the similarities with other therapy groups.

A constant theme of this group was a marked inability to handle aggression and its destructive implications. This was spelled out in the interactions within the group, and its unadorned quality often threatened the survival of the group. The aggression was handled by some members through psychosis, by others through depression and somatization. Ultimately it led to the Halls' and subsequently to the Davidoffs' leaving the group. The last nine months of meetings were attended by only the Rifkins and the Olans.

As is characteristic of parent groups, subjects for discussion were often approached by displacement of the problems onto the children. At first, members would discuss their difficulties only in this way. Over the course of the meetings they were increasingly able to talk about themselves directly and to accept the leader's clarifications about similar concerns being present in members of the group.

Distrust in the early meetings centered about fears of exposure. Related to this fear were the parents' intense guilty feelings about their children's illness. The members told how they rationalized the children's problems and followed this by intellectual discussions about the causes of mental illness. Most members supported theories

[9] Slavson, S. R.: *A Textbook in Analytic Group Psychotherapy*, New York, International Universities Press, Inc. 1964.

of chemical imbalance, except for the Rifkins who felt that the
environment was crucial. Mr. Hall expressed the conflict for the
groups:

> "This blaming routine is nonsense. It is ridiculous to blame our-
> selves. . . . It certainly is rough on a person if he is not able to
> contend with the outside world, but the world is rough. . . . You
> can get frustrated and short-circuited if you start blaming yourself all
> the time."

Mr. Rifkin agreed in part but added, "If you blame yourself, you
can do something specific about it and that might be good." This
interchange was the first of many expressing intense guilt that the
members were experiencing about their children's difficulties.

The dangers of the aggression that members felt were elaborated
early in feelings of how children can be hurt if they played with
other children. The members described their extreme protective-
ness, sheltering, and infantilization of their children. Mrs. Rifkin's
comment was characteristic:

> "Ernest was tired at home too, but he likes to be in his own bed in
> his own room and turn off the TV when he wants to. And I like it
> better too. I like to care for him as if he were an infant. After all, he
> is our only child. Each night when I get up, I glance into his room
> to see that he is all right."

Mrs. Olan talked about having left Linda at home for the first
time the week before while she went on a weekend vacation with
her husband. When they came home and brought Linda back to
the hospital, "she broke down and cried and made me feel awful . . .
it was not worth going away to have to come back to such a situation."

The members could gradually acknowledge the amount of discord
within their own family with the help of the leader who underlined
disagreements in the group. This led them to wonder if this was the
reason they had been selected for membership and also solidified a
common ground. Mrs. Olan said,

> "Linda is a problem, but the real problem is us. Last week we talked
> about discussions and disagreements. It seems like everything we
> talk about my husband and I disagree. If I say something is black,
> he says it is white. . . . This is definitely a problem in handling
> Linda, and of course she is well aware of the differences. . . . How
> do you find a compromise when there isn't any? The doctors won't

tell us how; they won't help us at all. . . . [to Mr. Olan] I want her
to come home even if you are not home because she certainly can't
come home while we are having such disagreements."

The comment by Mrs. Olan that the doctors did not help her-
alded the issues of the next five meetings. Mounting anger at the
leader gradually led to the emergence of psychotic defenses and
finally to regression to oral passivity. (An early discussion centered
around students who worked hard, but had teachers who gave
little.) Increasing complaints appeared about such things as the
leader not scheduling the meetings for a later hour in the evening.
During this time Mrs. Rifkin missed a meeting because of surgery
for a benign tumor. Mr. Hall became the most vocal member; he
described an experiment with guinea pigs and, when the leader related it to feelings about him and the group, he flushed, banged his
fist on the table, and said, "Put guinea pigs in quotes. It doesn't
matter what you call it, just forget it." Toward the end of the meeting when the leader made another comment, he replied, "You're
off your rocker." At the beginning of another session, he entered,
turned to the leader, and said, "Well, what's your problem tonight,
doc? Maybe we can help." The culmination occurred in the following meeting when Mrs. Rifkin entered in a rage stating that she
had heard from a non-group mother of an adolescent that the group
members disagreed. This meant to her that the leader was leaking
information. Mr. Hall was silent, and when Mrs. Rifkin asked him
to "bang on the table for me after every sentence," he revealed that
he had made a promise to his wife that he would be quiet. From
that time on, he was a model member, agreeing with and praising
every statement the leader made.

This series of meetings ended with the group's depression, summarized by Mr. Rifkin, "We can't change what the doctors do, only
what we do." The depression was accompanied by the emergence
of much oral material:

Mrs. Olan: I used to bring Linda ice cream, fruit, frappes, just to
get her to eat since she would not eat at all when she first came in.
However, after she gained the first twenty pounds and I saw there
was no end to it, I stopped bringing her things. Now my husband
says I'm to blame. Now she can't lose weight.

Mr. Rifkin: When Ernest was an infant, the cleaning man asked me
how it was that I had to have my clothes cleaned every week and

why they would get so dirty. I told him that Ernest was fed so much
that he could not take any more and would constantly throw up all
over me. . . . I frequently say that the past makes no difference, but
here we are at this stage of Ernest's life, and things are still just the
same as far as feeding goes. . . . My first statement when I came in
tonight was, "Have you seen Ernest and has he eaten."

Anger, alternating with depression and fear of exposure, continued. Anxiety during this period was high, manifested in most
members by tardiness and fear of talking because someone could
get injured. Mr. Olan said, "I get threatened before the meeting
that I'll be exposed when I come here," and his wife told that he
referred to the evening of the meeting as "his ulcer night." Mrs.
Rifkin reported an incident in which Ernest told her that "a boy
jabbed a girl with a pencil. . . . Ernest said he would like to punch
the boy, but he is afraid to do so." The depression which followed
such meetings was related by the group to their talk of family disagreements. All the couples revealed that they avoided conflict
within the family as well as in the group by turning off their participation. Mr. Hall began to talk with increasing emphasis, and at
times almost frenzy, about his need for internal controls, how easily
he was hurt, and how shaky his defenses were. He spoke of being
able to blot out anything he did not want to hear. Mrs. Rifkin said
she did similar things with her husband; "My medical doctor said I
simply could not have my husband upsetting me, so when he acts
like this, I simply close my ears." Mr. Hall continued, "But if someone disagrees with me, my attitude is I feel the poor devil is
wrong . . . I'm polite to everyone." Mr. Rifkin retorted, "You've
not shown any of that here."

The avoidance of specific details of members' problems was evident during this time. On one occasion Mr. Hall asked, "Well,
what is *your* problem, Brother Davidoff?" Mr. Davidoff replied,
"I've got plenty of problems," but the Halls quickly countered with,
"We took Sandy to Maine for the weekend; it was a wonderful
escape." It was during that meeting, which had occurred after a
two-week lapse due to a holiday, that Mr. Olan told of having a
mild coronary since the last meeting. When he said that he had had
bad news, Mr. Hall commented softly, "Me too," but this went un-
noticed. The hopelessness and helplessness was compounded by the
Olans' announcement that Linda would have to leave the hospital in

three or four months because she had been there for two years. The group was shocked and asked if the staff was giving up on her.

A crisis occurred a week later when the leader was unexpectedly absent because of illness. The members talked of the "dog-eat-dog" attitude of the outside world and the anger in their children. For the first time the Davidoffs could acknowledge their family strife, Mr. Davidoff turning to his wife and saying, "Go ahead and scream; show them how you do it." The group agreed that their problem was yelling at home and being nice in front of strangers. Mr. Hall reflected the danger implicit in closeness in his comment:

> "That's what I mean about the guys who fish and hunt in the Yukon: they are shut in quite a bit and all together. Frequently they get what we call cabin fever. This happens to a lot of guys like this. One guy wanted to saw a boat in half because he was so angry at the other people."

Just before the end of the meeting he revealed to the group what had been upsetting him for the past few weeks; "I've been a mess in business. I've turned to the hills, took the hounds, and was gone three or four days."

This series of interviews was culminated by Mr. Hall's serious heart attack several hours after the meeting. Mrs. Hall 'phoned the leader and decided not to attend the meetings herself. The Halls did not return to the group, although Mrs. Hall joined another several months later. The group handled the news by trying to protect Mr. Olan and not talk about it. There was also concern about the leader's health since he had missed the last meeting. The leader had to work hard with the group for over a month to help them acknowledge the impact of the loss. During that time, Mrs. Davidoff went to the hospital for the biopsy of a breast lump which turned out to be benign. The group joked about whether the meetings were too much of a strain on the members. Mr. Davidoff said, "If it's not one thing, it's another—mental illness, heart attacks, cancer." Later he told the story of a large family in which one member killed another and got three years for manslaughter. Mr. Rifkin, in this period, spoke of Mr. Hall: "If he was closer to us, perhaps we could feel more, but no matter how sick he was, he still was a pain in the neck. I feel sorry for him. He was completely without defenses."

The next several months was dominated by a new problem: a manic phase of Mr. Davidoff's illness, followed by depression, and, ultimately, with the Davidoffs dropping out of the group. The change in Mr. Davidoff occurred toward the end of the period of discussion about Mr. Hall's sickness. From his silent position, he became rambling and finally blurted out,

> "I had a nervous breakdown. I spent ten months at a state hospital just last year. I never told anyone. Now I can tell you. I can tell you all kinds of stories. You think you have troubles. I was in a . . . . . state hospital. There were naked people running all around, and people shitting on the floor."

Mr. Davidoff continued in this manner, and the group was stunned. Finally Mrs. Davidoff shouted, "Stop that! Stop that vulgarity!" With support from the leader, the group could help Mrs. Davidoff see that she was overreacting and set some limits on her husband's behavior. But the members were primarily overwhelmed by this experience. The most vocal member was Mrs. Rifkin who could only talk about it when Mr. Davidoff missed a meeting or was late. She felt that if Mr. Davidoff were mentally ill, then his language was excusable, but, if he was not, he was just vulgar. The leader attempted to get her to discuss this more directly with Mr. Davidoff, and this she certainly did, saying, "If you are cheap and vulgar because you are mentally ill, that's an excuse, otherwise, there's no excuse." This was greeted by stunned silence and an attempt by the other members to support Mr. Davidoff. Gradually, over another month, Mr. Davidoff became increasingly depressed, received little support from the group, and did not return. Mrs. Davidoff attended a while longer and also stopped. Attempts by the leader to get them to attend were unsuccessful; Mrs. Davidoff stated that she felt the members did not want them.

During the last nine months of the group the Olans and the Rifkins were regular, faithful members. Anger and depression continued as the main theme; however, the leader was more successful in helping the members get some distance from it, viewing the way they handled anger as a problem. They talked with appropriate sadness about Linda's leaving the hospital, her short stay at home, her rehospitalization at another institution, and her rather rapid deterioration. Gradually in the final weeks the members could acknowledge the importance of the group to them, and the feeling that their work together was really just beginning. Mr. Olan, who was most vocal about his indifference to the group, was tearful and so overwhelmed that he held a bottle of nitroglycerine tablets in his hand throughout the last meeting.

DISCUSSION

Although the members of this group were not chosen on the basis of their own personality problems, the primitive quality of the meetings implies severe psychopathology in most of the members. The evidence presented suggests that they had serious defects in their ego structure. Their difficulties were most manifest in the way they handled aggression, that is, by summoning primitive avoidance mechanism and ultimately showing impaired adaptational behavior. Their psychopathology coincided with the seriousness of their children's disorders, two of whom were acute schizophrenics and the other two latent schizophrenics.

Concerns about agression are common in therapy groups; however, the vicissitudes of aggression in this group were unique. Not only were the members' aggressive fantasies frightening to them and poorly defended against, but the way in which they interacted with each other reinforced the dangers of such aggressive thoughts and feelings. Their verbal attacks on their fellow members were often vicious. Their avoidance maneuvers in the group not only attempted to protect them from the threats implied in their fantasies but from the destructive ways which they used in reality to deal with other members.

Common defenses in the group were denial, projection, and distortion, manifested in times of group stress. These crises occurred as a result of increasing anger at the leader for not fulfilling their wishes to be protected and fed, and in response to illnesses in some of the members, i.e., as a result of relative deprivation and loss. At other times, more integrated defenses were maintained, but there was a fluid movement to the more primitive ones under severe stress. However, the theme of avoidance and escape was frequent.

Depression sometimes followed awareness that their primitive wishes were not going to be gratified. The depression was accompanied by a longing for food and the feeling that gratification prevented the danger of a never-ending void.

During the periods of increasing anger and depression, the amount of somatic illness within the group was impressive. Two of the men developed symptomatic coronary artery disease, one requiring hospitalization. Mr. Hall's serious myocardial infarct occurred in the setting of a business failure, the absence of the group leader, and the emergence in Mr. Hall of increasingly primitive aggressive fantasies. Two of the women were hospitalized for removal of benign tumors. The focus of the members on their bodies can perhaps explain their discovery of and concern with these lesions at that particular time.

The members' fears about their aggression in the group paralleled the parent-child interaction at home. Our impression is that the following sequence frequently occurs. The aggression which the parent or parents experience and find overwhelming is projected onto the world which is then viewed as a dangerous, hostile place. Their child too is seen to be in this vulnerable position which they themselves feel. He is then protected by them from these projected dangers by an infantilized relationship with one or both parents. This kind of relationship tends to reinforce and perpetuate the symbiotic ties and ill-defined ego boundaries between parents and child.

This formulation implies that the psychotic process in the child will tend to remain unmodified as long as the parents' aggressive fantasies are feared and defended against in the way described. In the therapeutic management of the child, much work is necessary to counteract the pull of the primitive ties which the parents attempt to maintain. If the adolescent plans to live with his parents after hospitalization, then the problem becomes more acute. This is especially true if the family psychosis is encapsulated in the relationship with the child.

Group psychotherapy with such parents can offer a means of interrupting and modifying this style of living through a corrective ego experience.[10] Such an experience consists in the working-through in the group of a trusting, gratifying relationship between the members and the leader so that conflicts inadequately solved can be reopened, be experienced affectively in the group situation, and settled in a more adaptive manner. As discussed above, the problems around aggression with these particular parents appeared rapidly. The group can provide the setting in which the anger can

---

[10] Semrad, E. V.: Long term therapy of schizophrenia. Paper read at symposium *Psychiatry in the Mid-Sixties*. Nov. 19, 1964, New Orleans, Louisiana.

be felt with increasing safety. The group experience in learning to bear anger and finding that it does not have the destructive potential feared can help open other avenues for its discharge. Hopefully, the experience would assist the ego in learning more mature and flexible defenses and free it so that it can function with increasing awareness of reality.

The leader's function is to establish the setting for such work to take place. Ultimately, his role as a model for identification is crucial if any major change will occur. He can demonstrate the flexibility of his ego, its ability to observe, bear anxiety, and handle other affects. This provides the model which the members imitate and eventually internalize.

It is difficult to evaluate changes in the members of this group. Half the members remained for the entire one and one-half years, and it is in these that some changes were evident. Both the Rifkins and the Olans became a little more tolerant of each other's anger and could talk about it without almost total disruption of the group. There was more empathy for the other members' problems and a greater ability to bear feelings of hopelessness about their own and their children's slow progress. Toward the end of the meetings, there were signs of the members' caring about the others as individuals. However, there is no clear evidence that these beginning changes in the group led to any significant modification in their relationship with their child.

Also significant was the relative inexperience of the leader who was early in his second year of residency when the group began. He was unprepared for the blatant, vicious quality of the aggression, and tended to permit the aggression to fulfill its dangerous potential rather than step in with the control and clarification that was needed. When he became more comfortable later in the course of the meetings, the group could work more safely and effectively. However, the early emergence of uncontrolled anger set the stage for supporting the distrust which the members brought in.

Although the group reported on in this chapter fell short of the therapeutic goals discussed, many issues were clarified and suggest that this method has considerable therapeutic potential. If the pitfalls described here are anticipated and overcome, group psychotherapy can become an important tool in the treatment of parents of severely disturbed adolescents.

PART V

Outcome

Several different studies of outcome—at time of discharge, six months after discharge, and a year after discharge—were done independently by members of the research team. The results of these studies were then compared, changes in the Cohort at the different points in time were measured, and the important question of predicting outcome was considered in depth.

CHAPTER 11

Evaluation of Patients at Discharge

The study of outcome for a group such as ours is a complex and multifaceted problem. Some of the questions which arise are: When should outcome be studied? Are we interested in results at the time of discharge from the hospital or results at one or more later times? Then, who should study outcome? Should it be someone familiar with the patient or at least with the patient's hospital records, or someone entirely unfamiliar with the patient's past? Thirdly, what variables should be studied? Should someone evaluating the outcome study only fairly obvious objective measures such as: Is the patient at work? Is he living at home? Or should there be an attempt to rate his status or his improvement in a more global and perhaps subjective sense?

The questions were not approached by a single methodical initial plan; in effect, several different studies of outcome were done

---

Based on work by Daniel Levinson and Bruce Sklarew.

independently. First of all, the patients were evaluated at the time of discharge by their own therapist, the person who knew them best in the hospital. Second, those who had been discharged were evaluated within a year after discharge by a single research social worker familiar with their previous records, who interviewed the parents usually in their own homes. The worker's ratings were mainly of objective findings, but she also rated global improvement and overall level of functioning at the time of follow-up. Third, a follow-up of the patients was done by two psychiatrists who interviewed them an average of one year and seven months after discharge. These doctors rated improvement "in the chief complaint" since admission and several aspects of the patient's level of functioning at the time of follow-up.

In this section, each of the follow-up studies, the methods used in gathering the information, and the results for our group of adolescents will be discussed. We shall also compare these various measures of outcome for the group as a whole. Finally, we shall be concerned with the question of predictors of outcome, or prognosis: the group will be categorized in a variety of different ways, and we will discuss what factors in the patient's early history, his illness, his appearance at admission, or his hospital course correlate with a good or poor outcome, as measured in our three outcome studies.

Methods of Assessing Patients at Discharge

We decided to utilize staff ratings as the primary method for assessing the degree to which the patient's condition had improved or worsened over the course of hospitalization. An effort was made to obtain for each patient in the Cohort ratings from three staff members: the patient's therapist (a psychiatric resident), the chief of service, and the head nurse on the service. Various difficulties were met in obtaining ratings from the chief psychiatrist and the head nurse on all patients in a given service. In the end, it was decided to make use only of the ratings by the patient's therapist, which were completed in forty-eight of the fifty-five cases. This procedure has the limitation that, without multiple ratings, we cannot determine the reliability of the therapist's ratings. It would have been preferable to have had two or more independent ratings by different staff members on each patient, or perhaps a single consensual rating made jointly by the staff members who knew him best. While recognizing the limitations of the present data, we may note that in most cases the resident had intensive experience with the patient both in psychotherapy and on the ward.

In assessing the patient's clinical change between admission and discharge, we obtained two types of ratings from his psychiatrist.

1. The Rating of Global Improvement

On a form filled out at the time of the patient's discharge, the psychiatrist was asked the following question:

How would you rate over-all change in this patient, including emotional growth, symptoms, and social adjustment?

Worse
Same
Slight Improvement
Moderate Improvement
Great Improvement

The advantage of this type of rating is that it permits the rater to weigh a host of clinical considerations. Since in many cases the patient has improved in some ways, remained unchanged in others, and perhaps gotten worse in still others, there are advantages to giving the clinician some latitude in arriving at an overall judgment of net gain or loss. At the same time, this type of rating has certain disadvantages. It is susceptible to the wish of the therapist to see at least some small gain in patients who have shown no gross improvement. It also does not indicate the particular ways in which the patient has changed. Accordingly, in addition to the global rating, we obtained the following series of highly specific ratings.

2. Ratings of Specific Characteristics at Admission and at Discharge, and Measures of Change

We developed an extensive questionnaire containing a series of variables to be rated by the psychiatrist for each patient in our Cohort. There are fifty-two variables representing ten areas of personality and behavioral adjustment. The formulation of variables was guided by the following considerations: (1) We sought to cover many aspects of the personality that are commonly included in the clinical assessment of illness and health. (2) The variables and their component categories are defined as concretely as possible and are anchored to observable behavior. (3) This is not a "symptom check-list" inventory; the variables deal in part with specific symptoms but they also deal with various aspects of ego development and social adjustment commonly involved in adolescent disturbances. (4) The ratings are usually defined so that one extreme represents greater psychological "health," the other, greater "illness."

Ratings were obtained of specific items grouped into the following general areas:

A: Socialization-Withdrawal
B: Symptoms
C: Responsibility for Behavior
D: Ego Strength
E: Sexual Identification
F: Hostility
G: Industry

H: Relationship to Family
I: Relationships in Hospital
J: Independence-Dependence

The psychiatrist was asked to do two sets of ratings on each patient, one for the patient as he appeared at the time of admission, the second at discharge. The Discharge (D) Ratings were made within a few weeks before or after the patient actually left the hospital. The Admission (A) Ratings were less consistent in this regard. An attempt was made to have them filled out quickly, but in many cases they were not done until the patient had been in the hospital for some time. These ratings are thus contaminated to some degree by the psychiatrist's postadmission experience of the patient. Although efforts were made to minimize possible error here, the variations in time of making the Admission Ratings must be acknowledged as a source of difficulty.

The first step in the analysis of the Admission and Discharge Ratings was a factor analysis, which was used to reduce the large number of individual ratings to a smaller set of primary components. Six orthogonal factors were derived. It was possible to construct Factor Scales providing relatively pure measures for five of the six factors. The five factors are:

Factor   I.   Poor control of inappropriate sexual behavior.
Factor II.   Psychotic withdrawal, minimal object relations.
Factor III.   Anxious, self-deprecatory, passive-dependent behavior.
Factor IV.   Assaultive-aggressive, hyperactive-labile behavior.
Factor V.   Rejection of authority and personal responsibility.

Each scale provides a relatively good estimate of the given factor at both admission and discharge. The factor scales can be used for three analytic purposes:

1. The patients' scores at time of admission give an assessment of their clinical-behavioral functioning when they entered the hospital. For our present purposes we shall not consider in detail the individual factor scales. Rather, we shall combine the scores on the five scales into a single measure, the *Overall Severity of Illness at Admission.* The higher this score, the greater the degree of the patient's psychological disturbance and maladjustment.

2. Similarly, by summing each patient's scores on the five factor scales at time of discharge, we obtain an *Overall Severity of Illness at Discharge,* an index of his clinical status when he leaves the hospital. This is our measure of level of functioning at time of discharge.

3. Finally, by subtracting the Admission from the Discharge Score, we obtain a measure of *Overall Change in Severity of Illness.* By this criterion, the patient has improved when the Discharge Score is lower than the Admission Score; his condition is worse when his score at Discharge exceeds that on Admission.

The *Overall Change Score* supplements the *Global Improvement Rating,* described above, as an additional basis for the assessment of improvement during hospitalization. Both measures are obtained from the patient's psychiatrist. The *Global Improvement Rating* is the psychiatrist's clinical judgment, based on numerous considerations intuitively weighted and combined, as to the patient's final gain or loss over the course of hospitalization. The *Overall Change Score* is derived statistically from a series of more specific and structured ratings of patient characteristics at time of admission and again at discharge. The net change is the difference between the admission and the discharge status.

FINDINGS

Our major concern here is to assess the *outcome* of hospitalization. From the procedures described above, we derived three measures of outcome, as judged by the patient's therapist at the time of discharge from the hospital. 1. *Severity of Illness at Discharge;* (measure of clinical status or level of functioning at discharge). 2. *Change* in *Severity of Illness;* (difference between Admission and Discharge Scores on the sum of the five Factor Scales). 3. *Clinical Change as Measured by the Global Improvement Rating.*

Let us briefly consider the data on each measure, and on their interrelations:

Severity of Illness at Discharge

The possible range of scores on this measure is 15-75, with a midpoint of 45. Higher scores indicate relatively severe intrapsychic and interpersonal difficulties; lower scores indicate the relative absence of such difficulties. For the sample of forty-eight cases on whom these ratings were made, the Mean was 48.4, the Standard Deviation 6.9, and the Range 35-61. Since the five component scales cover a wide range of psychological functions and areas of adjustment, we would not expect to obtain many scores at either extreme of the possible range. For the purposes of rough classification, we may divide the sample into three groups as seen in Table III. Clearly, some patients were quite ill at discharge. In a few cases "discharge" actually meant transfer to another hospital; in many others the decision to discharge a patient from the hospital involved the clinical judgment that he was ready to resume life on the outside, and obviously did not require that he be free of disturbance in the opinion of his therapist.

Change in Severity of Illness

This score, it will be recalled, is the difference between the patient's score at Discharge and his score at Admission, on the set of Factor Scales. The higher the Change Score, the greater the overall improvement (or, more concretely, the greater the decrease in Severity of Illness). Thus, a score of 0 denotes no change; scores above 0 indicate improvement, those below 0 indicate a change for

TABLE III

Severity of Illness

Severity of Illness at Discharge	Scale Scores	Number of Cases
High	53-61	14
Moderate	45-52	20
Low	35-44	14

TABLE IV

Change in Severity of Illness

Change in Severity	Scale Scores	Number of Cases
The same or slightly worse	−7 to 0	16
Slightly improved	1 to 5	21
Moderately improved	6 to 15	11

the worse. For the forty-eight patients on whom these scores were obtained, the mean was 2.4, the standard deviation was 4.8, and the range was −7 to + 15. On the average, then, patients showed a slight degree of improvement on this measure. Using three gross categories for purposes of classification, we obtained the results seen in Table IV.

Global Improvement Rating

In this rating, as we have described earlier, the therapist is asked to give an overall intuitive judgment regarding the degree of clinical change shown by the patient over the course of hospitalization. For the five rating categories, the distribution of the forty-eight cases is shown in Table V.

By this criterion, then, twelve patients were the same or worse, nineteen were slightly improved, and seventeen showed moderate or great improvement. This finding is similar to that obtained by the Change Score, just noted, where the corresponding frequencies are 16, 21, and 11, respectively. The main difference is that the Global Improvement Rating gives a somewhat more favorable picture of treatment outcome, especially in the number of patients seen as considerably improved. It may be that, in making the intuitive global evaluation, the therapist validly used evidence of subtle improvement not covered in the more structured, descriptive ratings. On the other hand, the global evaluation may also permit expression of the therapist's wish to see overall improvement even when

TABLE V

Global Improvement Rating

Worse	1
Same	11
Slight improvement	19
Moderate improvement	14
Great improvement	3

concrete evidence is lacking. We obtain a correlation of + .39 between the two measures of improvement. This correlation, while statistically significant, is not large in an absolute sense. It suggests that the two measures are only partially overlapping.

In addition, we find the measure of *Severity of Illness at Discharge* correlates + .31 with the *Change Score,* and + .38 with the *Global Improvement Rating.* We thus find that, not surprisingly, patients showing a better level of functioning at discharge tend to be seen as having made greater improvement in the hospital. At the same time, *Level of Functioning* (Discharge Score) is partially independent of degree of improvement. Both types of measure are useful in assessing the outcome of hospitalization.

In the analysis to be reported in the chapters that follow, we shall use two indicators of outcome at time of discharge. First, the *Discharge Score,* which refers to the patient's severity of illness (or, conversely, his adequacy of psychosocial functioning) at discharge. Second, we shall rely upon the *Global Improvement Rating* as a measure of the degree to which the patient benefitted clinically from hospitalization. We select this clinical rating in preference to the Change Score on the grounds that it is valuable to have a measure allowing full sway to free clinical judgment and that the Discharge Score provides an alternative, more controlled measure of outcome.

We turn next to the study of outcome as assessed by two independent follow-up methods after the patients had a period of readjustment following discharge. We shall then explore the relationship between outcome in the follow-up period and outcome at discharge.

CHAPTER 12

Social Work Follow-Up, Six Months
After Discharge

The transition of mental patients from the hospital milieu to home, occupation, and outside community can be equated, in terms of results of hospitalization, to the concept of the recuperative period now well established in public health as a crucial factor in recovery.

In an effort to examine the kind of transition our Cohort made from hospital milieu to community, a questionnaire and a recording form were devised by the project's research social workers to evaluate the social adjustment of each individual member of the Cohort six months after discharge.

Who Was Interviewed and How

Social service postdischarge information about the Cohort was, for the most part, obtained by a personal interview with an adult member of the adolescent's family. A letter on hospital stationery was sent to the prospective informant no sooner than six months after the patient had left the hospital, requesting an interview at a specified time and stating the research nature of the proposed meeting. In the event the designated arrangement was inconvenient, the relative was asked to call or write the social worker to plan a meeting at a different time.

Fifty-one parents were interviewed: forty-five in their home, office, or elsewhere, five by telephone, and one by mail. Two relatives refused to be interviewed, and two could not be located. All but four of the interviews took place within a six- to twelve-month period after the patient's discharge. In four cases, unavoidably, more than twelve months had elapsed, but the interview was

---

Parts of this chapter appeared in *The social adjustment of adolescents discharged from a mental hospital.* Weiss, T. and Glasser, B.: Mental Hygiene, 49: 378-384, 1965.

directed to elicit information specifically about the period six to twelve months after discharge.

The interviews were structured to obtain information about the patient's adjustment to the family, to his studies or work, his social activity, feelings about his peers, and use of leisure time, and each patient was rated according to current level of functioning and overall improvement as compared to his condition at the time of admission.

LIVING ARRANGEMENTS AFTER DISCHARGE

At the time of the research interview, thirty-two adolescents were living with their families, generally in decent neighborhoods and physically satisfactory homes. Of the nineteen patients interviewed who were not living in the parental home, ten of the twelve who had been transferred to another institution at time of discharge were still institutionalized, four adolescents who had returned home at discharge had been reinstitutionalized (two of these were hospitalized, a third was in prison, and in the fourth in a special treatment center); two girls had married since discharge, one unmarried girl who had become pregnant during her hospitalization was in a maternity home, one boy was in the army, and one boy was living with his grandparents.

CONTINUATION OF PSYCHIATRIC TREATMENT

Eighteen of the thirty-five members of the Cohort who had been discharged to their homes had continued in therapy at MMHC as out-patients for various lengths of time. Two others in this group refused out-patient treatment, and fifteen were not offered continued treatment, although they were told further help would be available if they wished it.

At the time of the research interviews, only ten of the Cohort were still receiving psychiatric treatment on an out-patient basis, and of the total group contacted, regardless of whether they were discharged by the hospital, left the hospital against advice, or were transferred to another hospital, less than half were involved in psychiatric treatment either on an out-patient or in-patient basis.

In only two cases were parents receiving professional help on a regular basis. In one case where the patient was referred for private therapy, the mother was continuing to see (on a private basis) the same social worker to whom she had been assigned when her daughter first entered the hospital. Both parents of the other patient were in treatment with a psychologist who expected to begin to treat the patient after a few more sessions with the parents. Only seven parents actually verbalized their need for help in dealing with their child or said that they were trying to find further help or social outlets for the patients.

ADJUSTMENT TO THE FAMILY

The majority of the relatives interviewed felt that the patient had not been able to adjust to family life during this transition period (see Table VI). They reported difficulties in the general area of adjusting to the patient's presence and concern with his or her mental stability. Some informants stated that the family had *adjusted itself to the patient's pathology* and had taken over the hospital role of caring for and nursing the patient.

SCHOOL OR WORK ADJUSTMENT

Fifty-one members of the Cohort were included in the follow-up. Twenty-nine were neither working nor going to school in the community; of these fourteen were at home and idle; two were at special treatment centers, and thirteen were institutionalized. Only nineteen adolescents were working or attending school. Thirteen of these nineteen were making a good adjustment, but six were not

TABLE VI

Adjustment to Family
(according to informant)

Adjustment	No. of Patients
Unknown	4
Well adjusted (gets along well with family members)	5
Fairly well adjusted (gets along fairly well with all or all but one member)	12
Skewed adjustment (family had adjusted itself to patient)	9
Not adjusted (does not get along with family members)	25
Total	55

TABLE VII

Work or School Adjustment

Adjustment	No. of Patients
Unknown	4
Attending school, working, or both; good adjustment	13
Attending school or working; poor adjustment	6
Not working or at school—at home	14
Special placement— school or treatment center	2
Institutionalized	13
Other*	3
Total	55

* One boy in the army and two married girls.

doing well at school or at work (Table VII). In three cases, one boy in the army and two married girls, the interviewer was not able to apply these categories.

SOCIAL ACTIVITY

Information about the use of leisure time and the quality and quantity of social activity was secured in forty-six of the fifty-one families contacted (in five instances the information received was judged unreliable). Sixteen of the forty-six adolescents participated sporadically in physical activities such as walking, bowling, and swimming, either alone or occasionally with others, and spent some time at spectator sports or on a hobby. However, only seven of the sixteen seemed able to strike a good or even fair balance between the amount of time they spent in physical activities, social intercourse, sleep, work, study, and watching television. The majority, according to their parents, either stayed up all night studying or watching television or "daydreaming" and couldn't get up in the morning, or they spent all their time doing one thing—be it studying, watching television, sleeping, or looking at a stamp collection—to the exclusion of everything else.

Six of the adolescents engaged in no social activity whatsoever, either at home or in the community, while an additional twenty-four confined their social activities to their family, hospital acquaintances, or a lone friend. Sixteen seemed to have a social life of some sort, twelve had been to some dances or out on dates, and four went out with the boys or the girls as a group, but again it was spasmodic for most of the sixteen (Table VIII).

RATING OF IMPROVEMENT

The social worker made two global ratings of each patient in respect to overall improvement and level of functioning. In the first, overall improvement, three categories were used: improved, no change, and worse.

The patient was rated *improved* if there were any signs of improvement since time of admission, regardless of current adjustment. One very sick patient, for example, was judged improved because after hospitalization she no longer struck her mother as she had frequently and violently before the period of hospitalization. The mother felt that this improvement made it possible for her to tolerate the girl, despite her other restricting symptoms, in the home.

If there were no signs of any improvement, the adolescent was judged *no change*. He was considered *worse* if, on the basis of a comparison between the hospital record and the interview content, his social adaptation was lower or his symptoms were more restricting (Table IX).

Over half of the group, 54 per cent, were considered better than they had been before admission. Thirty-eight per cent were judged worse or the same as before hospitalization.

TABLE VIII

Social Activity

General Level of Social Activity	No. of Patients
Unknown	9
Has heterosexual relationships	10
Has group of friends of same sex	4
Has one friend and acquaintances	2
Has one friend only	6
Associates with acquaintances	6
Sees friends made in hospital only	6
Confined to family	6
None	6
Total	55

TABLE IX

Rating of Improvement

Rating of Change in Patient Since the Time of Admission	No. of Patients
Unknown	4
Improved	30
No change	10
Worse	11
Total	55

RATING OF LEVEL OF FUNCTIONING

In the second overall rating—level of functioning—the social workers rated the degree to which an individual fulfills the normative social expectations of behavior. Four categories were used: Good, Fair, Poor, and Institutionalized. These categories involved a summary of the patients' rating on precoded recording forms in the following four areas: (1) relationships in living situation, (2) social relationships outside the home, (3) productive life at school and/or work, (4) interests or use of leisure.

Good implied that the adolescent, if still attending high school was living with his family; if working, living at home or with contemporaries; if married, living with his spouse; and that wherever he was living, there be little contention between himself and those who shared the residence. The minimum requirement for outside activities was evidence of some group activity, a relationship with one or more contemporaries, and an interest which could be exploited during solitary leisure. If there was any behavior which deviated from the above, the patient would be rated *Fair*. To be rated *Fair*, the adolescent had only to be making some attempt to be productive. Those who did not qualify for categories 1 or 2 were rated *Poor*.

The question of home and community adjustment for those adolescents institutionalized at the time of the follow-up study is of course not meaningful. Several had been home for a time after discharge from MMHC. It is evident from the fact of rehospitalization within a short time that the family and patient found the experience tumultuous and intolerable.

Table X presents the gloomy picture of over half of our Cohort, either institutionalized six to twelve months after discharge or in homes they had turned into small psychiatric institutions by their restricting symptoms. Only one relative (the mother of the only patient who was rated in the *Good* adjustment category) was able to convince the interviewer that the transition period had indeed been fairly smooth.

CONCLUSION

Six to twelve months after discharge, only one patient was rated in the *Good* adjustment category in the judgment of the research social workers. Since the majority of our Cohort came from intact family units, were housed in middle-class homes in decent neighborhoods, and returned to their homes and families after discharge, it would seem that something more or other than a home environment is needed for adolescents during their convalescent period after hospital discharge.

At the time of the research interview, almost all parents reported difficulties in the general area of adjusting to having the patient in the home and coping with his behavior and symptoms. Yet only three of the parents and ten of the children were receiving psychiatric help. It is our conviction that a strong, stable aftercare program, with social worker, nurse, and doctor available to deal with crises as they arise, is crucial to a good transition from hospital to home.

CASE STUDIES (*continued*)

Patrick. According to Patrick's father, who preferred an office interview to a home visit, Patrick was doing very well and had "gone a long way." He had calmed down considerably, no longer threw things, and got up mornings, without quite so much of a struggle as formerly, in time to get to high school. Father complained that Patrick smoked too much, but presumably parents and

TABLE X

Level of Functioning

Level of Functioning	Number
Unknown	4
Good	1
Fair	19
Poor	16
Institutionalized	15
Total	55

Patrick were making a fairly good adjustment to living together since Patrick's discharge from the hospital.

The family moved to a three-room apartment in a better neighborhood, and now Patrick was no longer afraid to do an errand as he had been previously because of his fear of the other boys on the street. Patrick had not made any friends at the present high school. Father implied that the reason his son had not had lasting relationships is that they had moved about a great deal. His school adjustment was "pretty good." He generally got home from school around 2:15, visited the MMHC, got home around 4:00, had a snack, and then applied himself to either the television or to his typewriter. He used his typewriter to write a little newspaper of current events of three or four pages with the assistance of another former patient at the MMHC. Father stated that Patrick was very interested in television, typing, writing, drawing, and hoped to go into the broadcasting field.

Linda. The family moved to a suburban community of new middle-class homes around the time Linda was transferred from the MMHC to a state hospital. Linda occasionally came home for the weekend to this six-room, attractively and comfortably furnished house where she shared a bedroom with her sister. Mother said that since it was a new neighborhood for Linda she had made no friends, and it was too far from their previous home for old friends to come to visit.

Mrs. O. considered Linda better. She had been on insulin shock at the state hospital which seemed to have made her more alert and aware of what was going on, but her idea of reality and mood remained unchanged. For example, she was interested in news of the family but was afraid that they were not really well and that mother was hiding disaster from her. She envied her sister's active social life and resented the fact that her sister was reluctant to take time from her activities to visit Linda in the hospital.

Linda had broken her wrist in the hospital, but mother did not bother to ask how it occurred because "they probably wouldn't tell me anyway." At this point, Mrs. O. seemed to have lost hope of Linda's recovery and was having difficulty dealing with her sorrow and with the facts of Linda's illness. She would have liked to have someone to talk with, but had been unable to see a social worker in the hospital to which Linda was transferred.

CHAPTER 13

Psychiatric Follow-Up, One to Two Years After Discharge

The fundamental orientation of this follow-up study was clinical, and the central source of information was an interview with the adolescent patient by a psychiatrist. The goal was to assess the patient's functioning over a wide range of life activities. Prior to each interview the psychiatrists studied the patient's record and the social worker's follow-up study where available.

The interviews, conducted by two psychiatrists associated with this research project, took approximately one and one half hours each and were held either at the MMHC, in the patient's home, or in another state hospital. In a few cases in which the psychiatrists were not able to see the patient himself, they employed telephone interviews with the patient, interviews with a close family member, and, when available, data from a psychiatrist treating the patient.

The two psychiatrists doing follow-ups saw the first six cases together and made independent formulations and ratings. They then compared the ratings and considered them to be in sufficiently close agreement to warrant dividing the remainder of the patients and having only one psychiatrist interview each. The interviews were conducted at a median time of one year and seven months after discharge. The psychiatrists' schedules made it imperative that all interviews be completed within a specific two-year period; therefore, two patients were evaluated while still at the MMHC. For the group as a whole, forty-three cases were judged by the research psychiatrists to have been followed-up satisfactorily with a complete interview; eight had incomplete follow-ups; and four were lost completely to this follow-up study.

Based on the work of Nicholas Avery and Anton Kris.

RESULTS

Objective Data

In terms of residence, 60 per cent of the patients resided in the parental home at the time of this psychiatric follow-up, 10 per cent were in boarding schools or colleges, 4 per cent were in homes of their own, 4 per cent were in other domiciles, such as the armed services, and 22 per cent were in mental hospitals. The group in the mental hospitals were almost all hospitalized for chronic mental illness. Two, as mentioned, were still at the MMHC. In terms of occupation, 24 per cent of the group were working full-time, 20 per cent were in school full-time, while 4 per cent worked or went to school part-time. The remainder were neither working nor in school. These facts are similar to those found in the social work six-month follow-up study (Chapter 12), except that more patients were working at the time of this second follow-up.

Insofar as treatment is concerned, 25 per cent of the group were taking medication. Forty-four per cent were in psychotherapy. Thirty-five per cent had maintained some relationship with a member of the MMHC staff. In 30 per cent of the cases, according to the patient, the families were getting some form of psychiatric help at the time of follow-up.

Ratings

The psychiatrists made five major ratings of each adolescent, one measuring improvement and four measuring different aspects of functioning at the time of follow-up.

Improvement

Three categories were used; improved, not changed, or worse. In each case the baseline for these evaluations was taken from the "chief complaint" of the patients at admission as rated by one of the research project psychiatrists (E.H.). This standard was used because of its relative uniformity compared to the statements in the patients' admission anamneses. Patients were rated "not changed" unless there was definite improvement or exacerbation in the chief complaint. Thus a patient may be described as "improved" despite much evidence of current pathology. No attempt was made to estimate the underlying problem. A few examples of improvement ratings are:

O.R., age eighteen, male. Chief complaint on admission: "Suicide attempt or gesture on day prior to admission." At follow-up there was no problem of suicide, and no other qualifying factor such as chronic hospitalization. This patient was rated *improved*.

B.K., age eighteen, male. Chief complaint on admission: "Sudden change from a quiet, studious boy to open rebellion." At follow-up he remained rebellious to an inappropriate degree, although not clearly worse. He was rated *not changed*.

M.S., age twenty-one, female. Chief complain on admission: "Increasing compulsive rituals." While already then described as "totally incapacitated," at follow-up she was not only incapacitated but her life was threatened by chronic malnutrition because of the rituals. She was rated *worse*.

Of the forty-eight patients for whom there was enough information to warrant a rating, 48 per cent were rated *improved*, 42 per cent were rated *not changed*, and 10 per cent were rated *worse*. It is interesting that the percentage of the group considered improved according to these liberal criteria was slightly lower than the percentage considered improved in the social work follow-up study.

Level of Functioning

The four measures of functioning at the time of the follow-up involved:

1. The patient's relationship with his family.
2. Relationship with peers.
3. Success in major occupation, either school or work.
4. Mental status.

Measures 1, 2, and 3 were rated Good (G), Fair (F), or Poor (P), while 4 was rated Good (G), Fair (F), Fair to Poor (F-P), and Poor (P). In general *Good* included normal and close to normal functioning; *Fair* included definite disturbance in functioning but markedly better than *Poor*. The rating *Poor* was given when the disturbance overshadowed any success in the area under consideration. The final rating was simply a listing of the rating for the four measures.

1. *Relationship with Family*

Good	21%
Fair	42%
Poor	37%

Good: A stable relationship, showing age-appropriate independence and demonstrating mutual respect and at least some affection.

Fair: Relationship clearly impaired. No attempt is made to assess how much of this might be attributable to the patient rather than his family.

Poor: The relationship is totally or preponderantly void of the qualities rated *Good.*

CASE EXAMPLES:

B.B., age nineteen, female. This girl described the dinner table as the "storm center," where her father was sometimes sarcastic. Although her parents wished her to go to church, she did not go and rationalized her rebellion. She paid for her own clothing, whenever possible, to be independent. Although she criticized her father, she espoused his values of idealism, ivory-tower intellectualism, disengagement from society, and his scholarly pursuit of minutiae. She respects her mother and planned to be a social worker (her mother's field), but felt she could not get close to her, though they were closer than before. Although there were certainly problems in family relationship, the patient was rated *Good* in this area.

B.M., age twenty, male. This chronically hospitalized chronic schizophrenic boy had no contact at all with his mother who was also hospitalized at a state hospital. Unable to get along at home, he saw his father only once a week. While his father still had hope and provided private psychotherapy, the patient was little more than a confused, passive bystander. This patient was rated *Poor.*

2. *Relationship with Peers*

Good:	19%
Fair:	28%
Poor:	53%

Good: At least one mutual, intensive, gratifying relationship with another person of the same age and sex. Relationships with other peers of both sexes are not grossly restricted although not necessarily intensive.

Fair: Clear evidence of gross restriction in some aspect of relationships with peers. Such restriction may be either that there is no intensive relationship or that despite one intensive relationship there is some gross restriction, as for instance a definitely impaired relationship with persons of the opposite sex. If there is one intensive relationship but the intensity is only in time spent together without the personal investment and pleasure of normal intensive relationships, that relationship is regarded as restricted.

Poor: No friends at all, or only superficial acquaintance with schoolmates or fellow workers, or, for those still in hospital, only superficial acquaintance with other patients.

CASE EXAMPLES:

R.R., age nineteen, male. This boy described one friend with whom he had a continuing relationship. They shared double dates, occasional friendly "tussling," and serious talks. He had other friends, went to parties and showed no gross inhibition or disorder in other peer relationships. However, he tended to be a "buddy" with girls and took a "little brother" role with them to avoid getting too close. He was rated *Good.*

W.D., age nineteen, male. While this boy had one friend with whom he spent more time than with others, their relationship was not intimate, but limited to driving to school together, where they chatted about different things. Other relationships in school and on the hockey team were friendly but distant. He had a steady girl friend, for whom he bought a friendship ring, but their relationship was described as platonic. This boy was rated *Fair.*

K.B., age twenty-one, male. While K.B. mentioned two friends by name, they live in another city, and he had seen only one of them once in the past year. They did not write. He had no other friends, though he worked regularly at an ex-patient club on their show. He had no dates or relationships with girls. This patient was rated *Poor.*

3. *Major Occupation*

Good: 42%
Fair: 2%
Poor: 56%

Good: Full-time, stable employment or school. No evaluation of the appropriateness of the job or performance is made beyond an assessment of whether it is full-time or stable.

Fair: This rating, used only once for this variable, signifies part-time occupation, school, without any other occupation.

Poor: Not employed or only transiently employed or in school. Patients in hospital received this rating even if they attended the hospital school or work in the hospital. Similarly, home tutoring was rated *Poor*.

No examples are given because this rating is self-evident.

4. *Mental Status*

Here an attempt was made by the rater to evaluate the patient's mental status in the interview directly. The raters considered three separate areas as follows:

A. Formal Mental Status (appearance and behavior, reality orientation, mood, specific symptoms)

B. Responsibility for Behavior (delinquency, sexual impulses, aggressive impulses)

C. Self (ambitions, interests, energy, initiative, self-evaluation and responsibility for self, awareness of others, capacity for mature, mutual relationships)

Final ratings of mental status were then made as follows:

Mental Status

Good	12%
Fair	23%
Fair to Poor	19%
Poor	46%

Good: No significantly pathology in any area, i.e., all three areas
           are rated *Good.*

Fair: At least one rating of moderate pathology, but no ratings
           of severe pathology in the three areas.

Fair to Poor: These cases rated *Fair* in area C but rated *Poor* in
           either or both of the other areas. The purpose of this
           rating was to distinguish those very sick patients who
           showed some personal characteristics that tended to
           differentiate their weaknesses from the patients rated
           Poor who were more enmeshed in their illnesses.

Poor: A rating of severe pathology—*Poor,* in either or both of
           areas A and B plus area C.

The following is an example of how mental status was evaluated:

A.   *Formal Mental Status:* A tall, moderately obese, malodorous
boy, was in urgent need of a shave and haircut, and was wearing
soiled, baggy trousers and a dirty shirt. Though pensive, his smile
reflected a mixture of self-consciousness and superciliousness. His
speech was clear and to the point, but his thinking verged on the
psychotic. He was very suspicious (and slightly grandiose) since
he expected to be imprisoned for his radical letters to school authorities and feared his files might be searched by the John Birch Society.
There was evidence of great anxiety—though not of delusion—as he
spoke of being prey to viruses and of the consequences of missing
a bowel movement. He was overconcerned with the wrongdoings
of others. His mood was dominated by hypochondriasis, but there
was no evidence of overt depressive affect or hypomania. He was
an angry young man with an excellent intellect going astray in a
fight with the authorities. There was considerable ritualistic behavior concerned with bowel movements, and he had to stay away
from bathrooms at other times for fear of overhearing sounds
connected with defecation. *Rating: Poor.*

B.   *Responsibility for behavior:* There was no evidence of delinquency or uncontrolled sexual behavior. Physical expression of
aggression was under satisfactory control, but he sent three vitu-
perative letters to the school authorities concerning supposed mis-
appropriations of school funds by the principal and was now
threatened with expulsion after being caught. He was carried away

by fantasies of leading social protest movements without sufficient regard to reality. *Rating: Fair.* (Not *Poor,* because not overwhelming pathology.)

C. *Self:* Full of ambition and energy, he was plagued by a very low self-esteem and did not accept his genuine scholastic achievements as significant. He had little tolerance for his own feelings and weaknesses and was thus *very limited* in his insight. He blamed his parents for his past illness. Very self-centered, he seemed grossly limited in mature personal relationships. His awareness of the feelings of others seemed poor, but he made great efforts to engage people in political debate at school and at his part-time job. *Rating:* Fair.

Final Rating: Fair to Poor.

The results are summarized in Table XI.

TABLE XI

Psychiatrists' Follow-up Study: Summary of Results

Improvement:	Per Cent of Cohort Rated:		
	Improved 48	No Change 42	Worse 10
Level of Functioning:	Good	Fair	Fair-to-Poor	Poor
Relationship with family	21	42	—	37
Relationship with peers	19	28	—	53
Major occupation	42	2	—	56
Mental status	12	23	19	46

Interrelations

Some interrelations between the four ratings of level of functioning can be noted:

Fifty-six per cent were rated *Poor* on two or more measures, and 74 per cent were rated *Poor* on at least one measure;

Seven per cent were rated *Good* on all four measures, and sixteen per cent were rated *Good* on three measures;

Twenty-one per cent of the evaluations showed ratings of both *Good* and *Poor,* demonstrating marked inconsistency of functioning;

Where relationship with family was rated *Poor,* virtually all other ratings were rated *Poor.*

The following relationships were found between the ratings of improvement and the various ratings of level of functioning:

Cases rated *Improved* were rated definitely higher on level of functioning than those rated *No Change*, who were rated strikingly higher on level of functioning than those rated *Worse.*

All cases rated *Worse* on improvement were rated *Poor* on all four measures of level of functioning.

All cases rated *Good* on mental status were rated *Improved.*

A few relationships were noted between the objective data mentioned earlier and the improvement and level of functioning ratings:

Residence in a mental hospital was associated with an improvement rate of zero and with very poor levels of functioning.

Residence at school or in one's own home (not parent's home) was associated with 100 per cent improvement; however, this included only a fairly small group. Full-time work at time of evaluation was associated with very high improvement.

Full-time school was associated with a high improvement rate and good levels of functioning.

Part-time school or work was also associated with a high improvement rate.

Aggression

Aside from the major evaluations involving ratings of improvement and of total functioning, the psychiatrists made a separate rating of aggression because they believed aggression was not adequately covered by the level of functioning ratings. The patients were rated only as inhibited, normally aggressive, or overtly destructive—the same categories used by the research psychiatrist (E.H.) in rating patients at admission.

Twenty-four per cent were rated inhibited, 50 per cent normally aggressive, and 26 per cent overtly destructive.

Adolescents rated normally aggressive were generally also rated as more improved and better functioning than the patients in the other two categories.

Conclusions

There was still a great deal of pathology present in the Cohort at the time of this follow-up study. Only 48 per cent were rated improved, even on the very limited criterion of improvement in the "chief complaint." This is actually slightly less than the percentage rated improved in the earlier social work follow-up study. A single figure cannot be cited for overall level of functioning since the psychiatrists felt that function in different areas was often uneven and could best be rated as level of functioning in four separate areas. However, the fact that 74 per cent of the group were rated *Poor* (severe pathology) in at least one of the four areas gives a general indication of the extent of disturbance.

These figures suggesting considerable pathology in the group form an interesting contrast with the fact that 78 per cent of the Cohort were living in the community. It is apparent that the community, which in most cases meant the patient's family, was able to accept rather serious pathology. This can be seen as encouraging proof that even quite ill patients can get along outside a hospital. However, there is a less encouraging side as well; in some cases it was the psychiatrists' impression that the families were actually perpetuating the pathology and interfering with their child's progress. In these cases some form of separation from the family, even if this meant rehospitalization, would probably have been helpful.

Among the interrelations considered, it is especially noteworthy that a rating of *Poor* on *Relationship to Family* was almost always accompanied by ratings of *Poor* on the other measures and with no improvement since time of admission. This suggests that for these adolescent patients, the first steps in recovery may be in the direction of improving their relationships with the family and that perhaps a poor relationship with the family actually prevents improvement in other areas.

CASE STUDIES *(continued)*

Patrick: This rapid-fire, matter-of-fact young man, whose conception of life was given only in circumstantial terms, expressed strong emotion for only one person, Jack Paar, whose television show he watched regularly. His family situation was very poor. He was overclose to his mother and was constantly faced with a degraded, ill father. Most of his very considerable energy went into work as a bookkeeper in a novelty company and a variety of minor activities with a lot of moving about. He did graduate from high school. Relationships were kept relatively distant. Diagnostic impression at this time was of borderline personality with well-established obsessional features rather than neurotic personality disorder.

Linda: A chronically psychotic girl, whose mental status included disorganization of thought processes and inappropriate affect. After combined electro- and insulin-shock treatments and phenothiazine in high dosage, she was on the chronic, disturbed ward, no longer in seclusion, but not able to assume ground privileges or make visits home. If there was any sign of hope, it was in the fact that she was still capable of expressing intensity of interest some of the time, but the overall view suggested hebephrenia and deterioration.

CHAPTER 14

Correlations Among the Measures of Outcome

The question arises of how well outcome measured in each one of these studies correlated with outcome measured in the others. Our chief interest was in changes in the Cohort at the different times studied. However, the three studies differed considerably in what questions were asked and in who asked them, so that these variables have to be taken into account in addition to the difference in time of follow-up. Thus differences in outcome may be related to the difference in interviewing technique and the different questions asked and may not necessarily mean a true change in the group over the time of the studies. Nonetheless, it may be interesting to examine some relationships between the three different studies of outcome.

Table XII gives the overall figure for improvement in the three studies. The social workers' and psychiatrists' follow-up results use the same categories and the results are in general agreement—there appears to be about 50 per cent improvement, slightly more in the first study and slightly less in the second. The results of the therapists' ratings at discharge are not so easily compared with the others but appear to show a higher improvement rate. Aside from possible optimism on the part of the therapists, it appears likely that the patients were indeed considerably improved at the time of

TABLE XII

Improvement since Admission

	Improved	No Change	Worse
Ratings by therapists at time of discharge	36*	12*	
Rating by social workers about six months after discharge	30	10	11
Rating by psychiatrists about eighteen months after discharge	23	20	5

* Seventeen were rated "moderate improvement," nineteen "slight improvement," and twelve "no improvement."

discharge, but that for many this was not a lasting improvement. We cannot compare results on *Level of Functioning* in this way since the psychiatrists did not give an overall rating of level of functioning.

Some specific correlations can now be examined to answer questions concerning agreement—i.e., were the same adolescents considered to be improved or functioning well in the three different studies?

Tables XIII and XIV show that the therapists' ratings of "global improvement" correlated only very slightly with improvement in the two follow-up studies. As we shall see later, this "global improvement" rating also showed poor correlations with a number of other variables; it appeared to be much less useful than our other measures.

It can be seen from Tables XV and XVI that the *Level of Functioning* (overall severity), measure derived from the therapists' study at discharge, correlates fairly well with level of functioning in the social workers' study and with improvement in the psychiatrists'

TABLE XIII

Therapists' Global Improvement
versus
Social Workers' Improvement

| | | Therapists' Global Improvement | | |
		Moderate	Slight	None
Social Workers' Improvement	Improved	12	11	5
	Same	1	4	3
	Worse	3	3	2

$$\chi^2 = 2.9$$
not significant

TABLE XIV

Therapists' Global Improvement
versus
Psychiatrists' Improvement

| | | Therapists' Global Improvement | | |
		Moderate	Slight	None
Psychiatrists' Improvement	Improved	10	8	5
	Same	3	8	4
	Worse	2	2	0

$$\chi^2 = 3.5$$
not significant

TABLE XV

Therapists' Overall Severity at Discharge
versus
Social Workers' Level of Functioning

		Therapists' Overall Severity at Discharge	
		Good	Poor
Social Workers' Level of Functioning	Adequate	6	1
	Fair	8	4
	Poor	5	9
	Hospitalized	4	8

$$\chi^2 = 7.36$$
$$(p < .10)$$

TABLE XVI

Therapists' Overall Severity at Discharge
versus
Psychiatrists' Improvement

		Therapists' Overall Severity at Discharge	
		Good	Poor
Psychiatrists' Improvement	Improved	16	7
	Same	5	10
	Worse	1	3

$$\chi^2 = 6.11$$
$$(p < .05)$$

follow-up study (since they have no single "level of functioning" measure). Table XVII indicates that the social workers' level of functioning measure was closely related to the psychiatrists' measure of improvement; thus if "level of functioning" at discharge is considered rather than the therapists' rating of "global improvement," there is fairly close agreement between all three studies.

It might be useful to try to compare the studies more closely in terms of some of the specific areas investigated. Table XVIII presents an overall correlation matrix for the ratings in the two follow-up studies. It actually consists of the results of 45 separate χ^2 tables, including Table XVII.

In addition to noting that the general agreement is good among the overall ratings (level of functioning and improvement), we might look at some of the specific areas which were considered by both the social work follow-up and the psychiatric follow-up. Al-

TABLE XVII

Social Workers' Level of Functioning
versus
Psychiatrists' Improvement

| | | Psychiatrists' Improvement | | |
		Improved	*Same*	*Worse*
Social Workers' Level of Functioning	*Adequate*	6	1	0
	Fair	7	4	0
	Poor	5	11	1
	Hospitalized	4	4	4

$$\chi^2 = 16.2$$
$$(p < .05)$$

though the questions they asked were not quite identical, three areas were definitely covered by both studies. These involved *adjustment at work or at school, adjustment with peers* (including social activities) and *adjustment to the family.*

The social work category "adjustment to school or work" correlates quite well with the psychiatric category "occupation," which in effect means the same thing. The relationship here is significant at the .05 level. The social work category "social activity" was compared with the psychiatric follow-up category "peer relationships," since these seemed to be very similar categories. Again, the relationship is significant at better than the .05 level.

However, the two ratings of adjustment to family correlate very poorly, at levels easily attributable to chance. This finding could mean that in many cases family relationships changed greatly in the period between the two follow-up studies. More probably the differences can be explained in great part by the fact that the social worker spoke to the family members while the psychiatrist spoke only to the patient. It is reasonable to suppose that the category "adjustment to family" is the one that might be seen most differently by these two categories of respondents.

We also attempted to relate some of the specific factors in the therapist's scoring of the patients at discharge with the later outcome studies. There were only two possibly significant relationships. Psychotic withdrawal at discharge was related to improvement as rated in the psychiatric follow-up in that those who were rated as very withdrawn were found to improve less. Also, there

TABLE XVIII

	Social Workers' Family	Social Workers' School or Work	Social Workers' Social Activity	Social Workers Level of Functioning	Social Workers' Improvement	Psychiatrists' Improvement	Psychiatrists' Family	Psychiatrists' Peers	Psychiatrists' Occupation	Psychiatrists' Mental Status
Social Workers' *Family*										
Social Workers' *School or Work*	0									
Social Workers' *Social Activity*	0	++								
Social Workers *Level of Functioning*	++	0	++							
Social Workers' *Improvement*	++	++	0	++						
Psychiatrists' *Improvement*	0	+	++	++	++					
Psychiatrists' *Family*	0	++	0	0	++	++				
Psychiatrists' *Peers*	0	+	++	0	0	++	++			
Psychiatrists' *Occupation*	0	++	0	0	0	++	++	++		
Psychiatrists' *Mental Status*	0	++	0	++	0	++	++	++	++	

Relationships between different ratings in the Social Workers' and Psychiatrists's Follow-up studies. ++ indicates a relationship significant at p < .05; + indicates a relationship significant at p < .10; 0 indicates no relationship at these levels of significance.

was a slight relationship, again barely significant, between therapists' rating of aggression and improvement as rated by the social workers. The relationship was in the direction of more aggressive patients improving less. The other specific factors rated at discharge showed no clear-cut relation to later outcome.

In general there seems to be a fairly good relationship between the major measures of outcome despite the difficulties in reaching agreement. With the exception of the "global improvement" rating by the therapists at time of discharge, all the overall measures of level of functioning and improvement correlate well with one another, as do the ratings by the different investigators looking at similar areas of functioning. The generally good correlations lead to the conclusion that the adolescents who were doing well at discharge and six months later also tended to be the ones doing well a year and a half later. In other words, there does not appear to have been a great deal of change in terms of which adolescents were doing well during the period following discharge from the hospital.

CHAPTER 15

Prediction of Outcome

We are now in a position to discuss the question of prognostic factors or factors related to outcome—in other words what characterizes the adolescents who got better as opposed to those who did not.

This question is important theoretically in allowing an eventual approach to a reasonable and perhaps heuristic scheme of classification and is also of great importance practically in telling us which adolescents can be expected to do fairly well with a treatment program similar to the one we have described and which ones might benefit, if at all, from a radically different sort of program.

In a situations where diagnoses are clear-cut, where we are dealing with a population suffering from several definite diseases, we would expect, of course, that the diagnosis would be one of the factors most clearly related to outcome. Thus, on a mixed medical ward including some patients suffering from pneumonia, some from myocardial infarction, and some from cancer, we would expect that the knowledge of diagnosis alone would lead us to a very good estimate of outcome or prediction of which patients would be doing well and which poorly a year later. However, diagnosis, according to formal psychiatric categories (A.P.A. classification) turns out not to be among the most useful prognostic factors, and therefore it is necessary for us to examine a large number of other factors we have available to determine which ones are or are not related to outcome. In fact, since we had suspected that diagnosis might not be a useful prognostic factor, one of the aims of the study was to devise various ratings of the patients on admission which might be more useful prognostically. These ratings were mentioned briefly in Chapter 3 and will be examined here in terms of their prognostic value.

We accumulated data on 25 demographic variables describing the patient prior to his illness; on 15 variables describing the patient's

Based on work by Ernest Hartmann.

illness and picture at admission, some of which were devised especially for their possible prognostic usefulness; and on 17 variables relating to the patient's course in the hospital (Chapters 2, 3, and 4).

The relationship between each of these 57 "predictor variables" and nine of the outcome variables discussed in the three outcome studies was determined using χ^2 contingency tables. Since this resulted in a total of 513 tables, several apparently significant single relationships would be expected by chance. Therefore in the interpretations, we have avoided pointing out single significant relationships and discussed instead the trend of relationships between a "predictor" variable and all of the outcome variables.[*]

PROBLEMS

Before considering the actual results, we must point out some relevant problems in several areas, from the collection of data to the interpretation of results.

The last four chapters described the various follow-up ratings which serve as our data for outcome. The data on the "predictor variables" derive from several different sources. Some of the "demographic" data comes from social workers' reports, while some comes from a series of informational forms filled out by each patient's therapist. The "time of admission" data and "in-hospital" data derive partly from ratings made by psychiatrists on our project (E.H. and H.C.) and partly again from forms filled out by each patient's therapist. The quality of these data of course is dependent on the care with which the data were obtained and the accuracy of notation and handling. The most problematic source of data was the form filled out by the therapists for this project. The therapists were asked to answer each item with care; however, there were a large number of questions, some involving aspects of the patient's past with which the therapist was not precisely familiar, and it is possible that the therapist occasionally made a guess rather than taking the trouble to obtain exact information. Every item on

---

[*] These variables are: "Global Improvement" and "Level of Functioning" from the therapists' evaluation at discharge; "Improvement" and "Level of Functioning" from the social work follow-up; "Improvement," "Relationship with Family," "Relationship with Peers," "Major Occupation" and "Mental Status" from the psychiatric follow-up study.

each patient could not be checked against independent sources; therefore it is conceivable that some error crept into the study at this point. We are reasonably certain that such error would be small, and there is no reason to suspect it would introduce a systematic bias in any particular direction.

We then had to face some problems in the analysis of the relationships of these data to outcome:

One problem is whether we can discuss outcome as a whole or whether we shall have to discuss one set of predictor variables related to outcome at discharge as rated by therapists, a different set of variables related to outcome six months later as rated by the social workers, and a third set of variables related to outcome as measured by the psychiatrists a year and a half after discharge.

Actually we can ask two questions:

1) Do the three sets of outcome measures intercorrelate well enough to permit the use of the concept of "overall" outcome?

2) Do single predictor variables correlate similarly with each of the three sets of outcome variables?

A perusal of the data convinces us that both questions can be answered in the affirmative. With one or two exceptions, which will be mentioned, there were good intercorrelations and consistent trends across the three outcome studies, so that we can consider the relationship of the perdictor variables to "overall outcome."

Another problem is that, as mentioned, outcome was rated in two ways in our outcome studies: as *improvement* since admission and as *status* or *level of functioning* at the time of evaluation. Do these constitute two very different outcome measures, and should they be considered separately? *A priori* we might have thought that this was indeed the case; that, for instance, some of the adolescents who had been extremely ill at the time of admission would have a lot of "room for improvement" and thus might be rated as very much improved at the time of the follow-up studies even though their level of functioning might be quite poor. However, one interesting aspect of the results is that this expectation was not fulfilled. In other words, the social workers' ratings of improvement correlated extremely well with their ratings of level of functioning, and the same was true to almost the same extent of the psychiatric ratings; thus, it appears that at least in these particular studies the adolescents who were rated as having improved at a particular time were also those judged to be functioning at a better level. Why this should be is not entirely clear; it is possible that the raters were actually rating only their overall impression of how well the adolescent was doing both when they claimed to be rating improvement and when they claimed to be rating functioning. However, it must be remembered that improvement was always rated against status at time of admission to the hospital, a time when all the adolescents were at a low level of functioning. Thus, a rating of improvement from their baseline status at admission would indeed show that the adolescents who were in general functioning best were also the ones who improved most from this temporarily regressed condition.

In any case, these results make it possible to discuss variables related to outcome as a whole, without having to differentiate between "improvement" and "adjustment level" outcome and in general without having to differentiate between the three different studies of outcome.

Results

Three sets of predictor variables, "demographic," "admission," and "in-hospital," are presented in Tables XIX, XX, and XXI, respectively. Each table lists all the variables in three columns according to whether the variable was (a) not at all related to the nine ratings of outcome; (b) weakly related to outcome, meaning that there was a trend in the indicated direction, but significantly related (p < .05) with not more than one of the nine measures of outcome; or (c) definitely related to outcome, implying a strong trend with significant relationships (p < .05) with at least two (and usually more) of the measures of outcome. We shall discuss briefly the factors that were found related to outcome and also some of the ones which were found *not* to be related to outcome although they might have been expected to have been related.

Demographic Variables

Looking first at the pre-hospitalization or demographic variables (Table XIX), we find that most of them, including age, religion, and so on, were not related to outcome. It is interesting here that sibling order was not related to outcome within this hospitalized

TABLE XIX

Variables Related to Outcome: Demographic Variables

Not Related to Outcome	Weakly Related to Outcome	Definitely Related to Outcome
Age of patient at admission	I.Q. estimate: higher I.Q. (+)	Early separation from father (−)
Religion	Father's education: less education (+)	Early separation from mother (−)
Sibling order	Temper tantrums (−)	Chumships during adolescence (+)
Education of mother	Previous psychiatric hospitalization (−)	Good object relations (+)
Family moves	Patient values religion (+)	
Grandparent living in the household		
Patient values idealism		
Patient values rebellion		
Peer leadership		
Peer participation		
Enuresis		
Night terrors		
Court record		
Previous drug therapy		
"Pathogenic Family"		
Social class		

+ = related to good outcome   − = related to poor outcome

group, although it was apparently related to hospitalization in that over half of our Cohort were first or only children. Neither enuresis in childhood nor night terrors in childhood nor a court record, all of which are sometimes considered bad prognostic signs, were related to poor outcome. In these contingency tables, only one variable was considered at a time. It is still possible that the presence of a combination of several of the factors taken together might have turned out to have prognostic significance.

Likewise, social class did not show any definite relationship to outcome in this study, although the results of some other studies might have suggested that such a relationship would be found. This was somewhat surprising, since our impression had been that the patients from middle-class homes somehow felt more comfortable in the hospital and found it easier to conform to the hospital's expectations. However, it must be remembered that all the adolescents received psychotherapy, and the abundance of staff insured that no one was neglected, as lower-class patients may have been in other studies.

"Pathogenic family" represents an attempt by one psychiatrist (H.C.) to rate each family on the basis of information in the chart.

This rating failed entirely in predicting outcome. Temper tantrums were weakly related to a poor outcome, as was previous psychiatric hospitalization. Probably a stronger relationship was not found with the latter because "previous psychiatric hospitalization" could have included anything from a few days to many years. I.Q. estimate was weakly related to outcome in that adolescents with higher I.Q. tended to do better. None of these relationships are especially surprising. Somehow, the adolescents having a father with poor education tended to do better than the adolescent with a well-educated father; we have no explanation for this except that one or two "weak relationships" will occur by chance among the number of relationships we studied.

In considering the four demographic variables definitely related to outcome, it is interesting that both early separation from the father and early separation from the mother were found to be bad prognostically. Adolescents with either or both of these factors in their background appeared to be functioning worse in the outcome studies. The two other variables, chumships during adolescence and good object relations in the past, were both related to a good outcome, as might have been expected; a poor rating on these variables may be a reflection of some illness already present in the patient's past history.

Evaluation at Admission:

Turning to the variables involved in the evaluation of the patient at admission (Table XX), we find that many more of these appeared to be related to outcome. It is striking that of the fifteen or so predictor variables investigated, diagnosis by the admitting physician was the worst predictor; in fact it was the only one in this group of fifteen that appeared to be not at all related to outcome. This may well have been because, as mentioned earlier, these admitting diagnoses were made by more than fifty different physicians, who may not have been using terms in exactly the same way. Nonetheless, this is an interesting finding.

Although the diagnosis made by the admitting physician did not relate to outcome at all, a diagnosis made on all patients by a single psychiatrist (H.C.) for the research project was found to be weakly related to outcome. Here a diagnosis of schizophrenia was related to a worse outcome than a diagnosis of "adjustment reaction" or "borderline," but the relationship was not very strong.

TABLE XX

Variables Related to Outcome: Variables Involved in Evaluation of
Patient at Admission

Not Related to Outcome	*Weakly Related to Outcome*	*Definitely Related to Outcome*
Diagnosis made by admitting physician	Diagnosis made by a single psychiatrist for research project. Schizophrenia ($-$) as opposed to adjustment reaction or borderline	Acute onset ($+$)
		Patient presents himself with symptoms or signs. Signs ($-$)
	Duration of illness: long duration ($-$)	Defenses against infantile object ties: regression ($-$) displacement or reversal ($+$)
	Previous therapy ($-$)	
	Precipitating event: clear-cut external event ($+$)	Handling of aggression: normal ($+$) inhibited ($-$)
	Present illness a reaction to adolescence ($+$)	Presents self to hospital: Neurotic ($+$) Withdrawn ($-$) "Normal" ($-$)
	Confused at admission ($-$)	
	Defenses against instincts: less mature defenses ($-$)	
	Primitive defenses structure ($-$)	
	Handling of sex: Normal ($+$)	

Let us turn to the variables in this area which were found to be good prognositc factors in the column "definitely related to outcome." First of all, the question of acute onset: an acute onset of less than three months from health to full-grown illness was definitely related to a good outcome. This is similar to what has been noted in a number of other studies, not only of adolescents but of mental illness in general.

The question of whether the patient presented with symptoms or signs is interesting; in this study presenting with signs was definitely poor prognostically. In other words, the adolescents who did not feel that there was anything wrong with them, who came in mainly because they were disturbing their environment, were often the ones who did worst. The category "presented chiefly with signs" includes most of the behavior disorders, but also many adolescents diagnosed schizophrenic.

The variable "defenses against infantile object ties," adapted from Anna Freud, turned out to be one of the best prognostic variables in this study. This involved ratings, made by one research psychiatrist (E.H.), of whether the adolescent handled his childhood object ties chiefly by displacement, by reversal, by turning towards himself, or chiefly by regression (Chapter 3). Thus this variable involves, in a sense, a measure of maturity in object relations. "Regression" was definitely worst in terms of prognosis, as would have been expected, whereas "displacement" or "reversal" were both related to a good outcome. It was rather unexpected that this variable would show better correlation with outcome, than, for instance, diagnosis, or duration of illness, which we had thought might correlate with outcome very strongly.

Handling of sex and handling of aggression as rated at admission (these ratings referred not only to the time of admission but to the entire adolescent period) both turned out to be related to outcome. "Normal" handling of sex and aggression was the best category in terms of outcome. "Inhibited" handling of aggression was definitely related to a poor outcome, but the case was not so clear with handling of sex. In fact this was one of the few instances in which the follow-up studies disagreed. A rating of "inhibited" for handling of sex turned out to be related to a good outcome in the social work follow-up but not good, in fact slightly less good than average, in the psychiatric follow-up. This is a rather surprising finding; it seems unlikely that the adolescents who were sexually inhibited at admission should be definitely improved as a group six months after discharge and then definitely worse again a year later. It is more likely that those adolescents who had originally been rated as the most sexually inhibited were by-and-large still the most sexually inhibited at the time of the follow-up studies; yet this same situation might look better to a female social worker getting her information from the parents than to a male psychiatrist talking to the patient himself.

Another variable that turned out to be a good predictor of outcome was "how patient presents himself to the hospital" (Chapter 3). Presenting himself as "neurotic," as a patient coming for help with certain troubles such as anxiety or depression, was associated with a good outcome. Presenting himself as "withdrawn" or as "normal" was associated with a poor outcome: the other categories—"panic," "rebel," and "mixed"—fell somewhere in between.

Briefly, some of the variables that were weakly related to outcome included a variable related to the maturity of the defensive structure and a variable concerning the classic Freudian defenses against instincts. These were related as expected in that more primitive defenses were associated with a poor outcome, but the relationship was not so strong as with the "defenses against infantile object ties." Again, as expected, duration of illness was related to a poor outcome, though not very strongly. The presence of a clear-cut precipitating event was a good prognostic sign; this has been a common finding in many studies of psychotic illness in general. A rating indicating that the present illness was chiefly a reaction to adolescence was likewise a good prognostic sign. This rating, as far as we know, has not been used in other studies. Apparently the group of patients who had been doing well prior to adolescence, and who clearly decompensated, usually rather suddenly, as a result of adolescence were able to readjust successfully, at least after a few years. It seems likely that these adolescents temporarily needed a sheltered environment to allow them to rebuild their adaptive mechanisms.

In-Hospital Variables:

Our main finding in the third large group of variables—those dealing with the patient's course in the hospital—is that there were hardly any variables that bore a definite relation to outcome (Table XXI). The only variable definitely related to outcome was "discharged to where?"; obviously discharge to another hospital (usually meaning transfer to a large state hospital) was related to a worse outcome than discharge home or elsewhere.

Some variables were found to be weakly related to a good outcome; these included "patient getting psychotherapy after discharge" and "patient spending a great deal of his time outside of the hospital working or going to school while still a patient." Both of these certainly might have been expected. It is interesting, however, that psychotherapy after discharge showed some positive correlation with outcome, whereas the variables dealing with psychotherapy in the hospital showed no relationship with outcome. This

TABLE XXI

Variables Related to Outcome: In-Hospital Variables

Not Related to Outcome	*Possibly Related to Outcome*	*Definitely Related to Outcome*
Length of sessions with therapist	Amount of supervision for resident therapist: more supervision (+)	Discharged to where: hospital (−) home or elsewhere (+)
Average weekly hours with therapist	Patient's longest status: longest status "outside" hospital" (work or school outside while still a patient) (+)	
Group therapy		
Drugs in the hospital		
Parents in group therapy		
Family visits	Psychotherapy after discharge (+)	
Day program	Length of stay: Longer stay (−)	
School attendance		
Participation in patient government		
Suicidal?		
Acting out?		
Parents seeing a social worker		

may be due to the fact that while in the hospital all adolescents received psychotherapy, and the question was only how much, whereas after hospitalization less than half received treatment and the question was either psychotherapy or no psychotherapy.

The amount of supervision received by the patient's resident therapist was positively correlated with outcome; patients whose therapists received more supervision did best at follow-up. This may have something to do with the excellence of supervised therapy, but it is also possible that the resident therapist asked for and received more long-term supervision for the patients who seemed to be "good psychotherapy cases." It is still somewhat puzzling, however, that amount of supervision bore at least some slight relation to outcome, whereas amount of psychotherapy (see below) did not.

The long list of variables that did not turn out to have any relation to outcome is quite striking. It is not too surprising that the number of family visits or patient's participation in school, in a day program, or in patient government should not be related to outcome. It is perhaps somewhat unexpected that neither the presence of suicidal attempts nor acting out was related to outcome; however, "acting-out" is an ill-defined category assigned by the patient's therapist on a wide variety of grounds. Really serious suicide attempts did not occur often enough to be related to outcome as a separate category; the "suicide attempts" include many attempts that were more in the nature of suicide gestures used to get help or to get attention.

It is quite surprising, however, that no in-hospital treatment variable—neither amount of psychotherapy, nor drugs, nor group therapy, nor social work with the parents—was related to outcome. Are we to conclude from the data that none of these treatments are of any use to hospitalized adolescents? This would be a possible conclusion, but not, we feel, the most reasonable one. Obviously, psychotherapy or drugs were not given to a random sample of the population; rather, drugs and relatively more psychotherapy were usually given to the patients who seemed to need it more—the sicker patients. Thus, it may well be that the treatments had a beneficial effect approximately great enough to balance this sampling bias; this may be especially true for drug therapy. Furthermore, as mentioned, all the adolescents who were in the hospital for more than a few days received psychotherapy in some degree; our variables relates only to receiving more or less therapy, which is influenced by a large variety of factors. This study certainly cannot supply any sort of evaluation of the efficacy of psychotherapy.

DISCUSSION

The findings are not entirely what we had expected. If, before this study, we had wished to draw a composite picture, let us say, of the adolescent we expected would do poorly as opposed to the adolescent who would do well, we would probably have used categories such as the following: the "poor-prognosis" patient would be an adolescent who had been ill for a long time, came from a "pathogenic family" and a lower-class background, and who had a diagnosis of schizophrenia, without an acute onset. In terms of the results of this study, we would now no longer be impressed principally by the actual diagnosis or by a supposedly "pathogenic family." We would characterize the adolescent expected to do poorly in our setting as a patient who had had separations from his parents early in life, had failed to make any friends during his childhood or adolescence, had a gradual onset of his illness, handled his infantile object ties by regression (returning to earlier modes of dealing with people), was inhibited in his sexual and especially aggressive activities, and then either arrived at the hospital in a "withdrawn" state or presented himself as normal ("nothing wrong with me").

The patient who could be expected to have a good outcome would be one who had had good object relations, did have friends during adolescence, was normal in sexual activities, and normal or active in his expression of aggression, and who handled his object ties either by displacement, turning his affections from his parents to friends, or by reversal, becoming angry and rebellious toward his parents, and then presented himself to the hospital with specific problems that concerned him ("I'm too anxious" or "I feel depressed"). If in addition to all this, he worked or studied outside the hospital while still a patient, made sure his resident therapist had plenty of supervision, was discharged from the hospital to his home, and continued in psychotherapy after discharge, his outlook would be excellent indeed!

It must be kept in mind, of course, that all these results refer to outcome after hospitalization in a particular program. We are not justified in generalizing these findings to all adolescents in all treatment settings.

However, we can say that at least in our setting, prognosis appears to depend on ego-functioning—on relationships with others, on the handling of impulses, on the ability to acknowledge difficulties and ask for help. This is not particularly surprising and agrees to a great extent with what we might consider an "intuitive clinical judgment." Yet in this study we have been able to *quantitate* and *rate* these clinically derived factors sufficiently accurately to allow a far better prediction of outcome than was achieved by the more usual diagnostic criteria.

PART VI

Conclusions

Adolescents can be treated on adult wards—after these years of study, there is no question about that. Questions do arise, however, that call for further study, analysis and clarification. Would some adolescents be better off in other treatment environments? Would all adolescents do better if placed in a general hospital ward with emotionally healthy adult patients? . . .

What would be an ideal hospital environment for mentally-ill adolescents?

CHAPTER 16

Meeting the Tasks of Adolescence in a Therapeutic Inpatient Program

The experience gained in studying and treating hospitalized adolescent patients on adult wards, which has been detailed in this monograph, has led us to consider how we could plan for an *ideal* environment, assuming adequate resources. The question is a pressing one, not only because of the growing numbers of adolescents admitted to mental hospitals—far outnumbering what would be expected from population increases alone—but also because the adolescent is so vulnerable to environmental influences of all kinds. A great many patients first admitted during their adolescent years have been living in our mental institutions for decades because of

Based on work by Gertrude Rogers and Milton Greenblatt.

the failure of treatment. We wonder whether proper therapeutic management in their first admission would have forestalled this chronicity.

It would be foolhardy to plan a satisfactory in-patient program without consideration of the *tasks of adolescence,* both generally and in relation to the unique requirements of each individual adolescent. We consider the tasks of adolescence to be:

1. Emancipation from early object relationships.
2. Reorientation to authority.
3. Achievement of a new identity.
4. Satisfaction of intellectual curiosity and the establishment of mastery over some challenging area.
5. Development of a stable set of values—a philosophy of life.

To become mature, the adolescent must make progress in all areas. However, the requirements for growth may vary considerably from one adolescent to another. There may be arrested or disturbed development in one or in many areas. For example, one individual may achieve considerable intellectual development, without parallel success in emancipation from familial objects. Another may make satisfactory progress in adapting to biological or social demands without much drive in the intellectual sphere, or he may delay for a long time crystallizing a set of enduring values. Progress begun in adolescence may continue for many years and there are often unresolved residua of adolescence in adulthood. Let us assume that the major challenges to adolescents are included in the tasks mentioned, if only to have a framework on which to base a discussion of the "ideal therapeutic environment." Our discussion must recognize that the tasks of adolescence cannot be conceived as separated elements of development but are necessarily interrelated in a total growing organism.

EMANCIPATION FROM EARLY OBJECT RELATIONSHIPS

This is a two-fold task: first, to resolve dependency and second, to change libidinal investments with regard to object, direction, and mode of gratification. In a word, old ties have to be altered or broken and new ones established.

With respect to resolution of dependency, we must remember that the sick adolescent has sick ties to parental or familial figures, and that often emotional deprivations have been so great that he has turned away from people or turned inward, with deep anxiety or anger mobilized whenever someone comes close.

Society, nevertheless, demands that the adolescent turn his attention from familial to extra-familial objects, that he develop a new balance between giving and receiving with more emphasis on giving, and that he replace pregenital primacy with genital primacy.

The sick adolescent cannot accomplish all this, even though his family may insist (at least verbally) that he become independent, even though his peers are negotiating with apparent ease the transition to adult life that frightens him, and even though he appreciates society's demands upon him. This inability is what upsets the adolescent, and leads to regression on admission to the hospital. The ties are broken and the hope of reconstructing better ones seems remote. He may suffer great turmoil and manifest typically adolescent regressive behavior by excitement, by striking out, by impulsivity, by noise, by unstable behavior, or by various degrees and kinds of withdrawal.

What is the optimum environment to aid the youngster in resolution of old dependencies and in reattachments? Several choices have to be made. Perhaps the first is whether to hospitalize him in an all-adolescent unit, in a unit with children, in a unit with adult patients, or in some combination of these. The literature is divided on this theme. It is doubtful that any one plan can suit the needs of every adolescent. Administratively it is simpler to organize programs where the age range of patients is narrow, as in an all-adolescent unit. Conversely, therapeutic planning for the diversified needs of all patients is more difficult when adolescents live in units with children or with adults.

Our preference was for adolescents to live in wards with adult mentally ill patients, but with a broad socio-recreational and educational program designed specifically for them. This not only approximates the situation in the world outside, but there is the additional advantage that the tendency to regress when faced with separation from familial figures seems to be less in the adult ward. Dietz et al.,[11] in a separate study under our direction, showed that in

---

[11] Dietz, C. J., Lott, W., and Glasser, B.; Transfer from all-adolescent to adult wards as a treatment measure, Submitted for publication.

twenty-four of twenty-seven consecutive instances of transfer of very disturbed adolescents from an adolescent ward to adult wards in a large mental hospital, the disturbed behavior improved decidedly or disappeared altogether. Moreover, there was no evidence that other abnormal behavior was substituted. On the adult wards there was less stimulation, fewer activities, and diversions than on the adolescent ward. There was also a sharp decrease in rivalry for the attention and affection of personnel; at the same time the adolescent seemed to enjoy a special "place" among the adults. Disturbed behavior was no longer rewarded by attention and imitation from others. The adolescent was more conscious of authority, and noted the conformity of both patient and staff to expectations of responsible behavior. Thus, living at least part time among adults may help the adolescent control his behavior and overcome the tendency to regression and fixation at levels of impulsivity and disorganization.

Another choice has to do with the participation of parents or parental figures in the treatment program. Mistakes are usually made on the side of inadequate involvement of parents. Clinical judgment will dictate decisions on visiting privileges, involvement of parents in therapeutic relationships, and/or in the socio-recreational life of the ward. A most interesting approach, usually under research auspices, involves parents and adolescents living together in hospital suites especially designed for intensive care and study.

Resolution of dependency requires not only an environment conducive to the formation of new ties but also the dedication of individuals willing to commit themselves to the task of forming long-term intensive relationships with the adolescent, giving him support and understanding, and imparting their belief in his ability to grow. Such relationships have to be sufficiently rewarding in the long run to permit the adolescent to relax his infantile grip on family members. In the course of such work, as we have indicated in Chapter 8, there is bound to be considerable anxiety and stress, sufficient to tax the patience and forbearance of all those involved. Although some patients may show heartening progress early, most adolescents whose illness has reached the depth of disturbance shown by our study population will need many months or years of consistent psychotherapeutic aid from at least one individual. Meanwhile, the adolescent will be strengthened in whatever area of life lends itself to strengthening, while waiting for deeper therapy to achieve its goal.

Continuity of staff and maintenance of support is as important in the follow-up period as in the inpatient phase. In training situations, where psychiatric residents provide most of the therapy, continuity of approach and philosophy should be emphasized to offset changeover from one resident to another.

REORIENTATION TO AUTHORITY

The ideal therapeutic environment will have to develop structure suited to dealing with the adolescents' struggles against authority. These struggles take many forms, overt or covert, conscious or unconscious, and the adolescent may commit his available energies partially or fully to overthrowing authority. The MMHC, like most small treatment centers with open wards and without security measures, had its limits of tolerance; thus, many adolescents who acted out violently were either not admitted or were admitted but later transferred to a large state mental hospital. If many adolescents are to be treated in the same environment, and yet have therapeutic management highly individualized, much planning is necessary to achieve both flexibility and consistency. One single environment cannot be optimum for all types of patients. Our findings indicate that an environment such as MMHC, based on permissiveness and freedom, had limitations in dealing with chronically antisocial and acting-out disorders. Any cultural "set" imposes difficulties for those who are marginal or alien to that set.

Authority as represented in the hospital social system can present a stronger, more consistent, more rational, and more benign aspect than was presented to the patient at home. Authority is implicit in the set of rules and regulations that structure life on the ward, and it should be interpreted daily, openly and therapeutically, by ward administrators, nurses, attendants, and other professionals. In the ideal therapeutic environment, the system of rewards and punishments, or limit-settings, has to be individualized to fit the patient's needs and level of tolerance. Then the staff has to stand fast against the adolescent's manipulations to undo or defeat the structure. Their ability to do so, as we have found in our study of staff attitudes, will depend partly on the extent to which staff members have resolved their own adolescent conflicts. Persistent efforts must be expanded to unmask the meaning and effects of the adolescent's manipulative behavior in a form that is easiest for him to recognize and digest, while any constructive attempts to adapt to the system are properly rewarded.

In the extreme case, the adolescent will be so committed to destroying his environment that an auxiliary ego will be necessary to supply controls during almost every moment he is in contact with ward society. Such a patient may require step-by-step rebuilding of his adaptive capacities before he can be allowed to be a member of a group. In the more usual case, the adolescent will attempt to exploit cracks in the authority front—differences of opinion, philosophy and therapeutic practice—so as to set one person off against the other. The importance of repeated discussions and understanding with respect to philosophy, method, and technique of the therapeutic staff relating to the adolescent is therefore obvious.

With alienation from parental figures, the identification vacuum will be filled by new interests and attachments. Here the hospital environment offers the advantage of a variety of relatively mature individuals of various ages, personality types, and work commitment with whom to identify. This aspect of the adolescent's development is fully as important as the resolution of parental ties. As positive identification begins to replace negative rebellion, he begins to resolve his conflict with authority. He comes to recognize that although authority may be firm and intractable on certain issues, it is also capable of being benign and understanding. This points the way to satisfactions in life that can be accepted without the necessity of overthrowing the social organization. Identification and internalization of new models begin to lay the foundation for a better synthesis between inner and outer demands.

As external emotional controls become internalized and testing of limits not so necessary, the adolescent moves toward moderation in emotional expression—expression more appropriate to the adult world. A further gain is improvement in his reality sense, for inner and outer reality have become more congruent. As these changes radiate throughout his personality, the way is paved for achievement of a new identity.

ACHIEVEMENT OF A NEW IDENTITY

Not only are there rapid and profound changes in the biological sphere during adolescence—in body size and shape, muscular and fatty distribution, and physiological activity, but there are also changes in body image, areas of sexual feeling, and energy output. The therapeutic environment has to meet the great need of adolescents for body mobility, exercise, and recreational activities, and set a framework within which appropriate ways of coping with libidinal drives can be encouraged and facilitated. Thus, a scheduled activities program, sports, gymnastics, and a wide variety of group recreational activities demanding vigorous expenditure of energy should be integrated into the overall treatment program. In addition, the therapeutic organization should provide opportunities for both sexes to mix together and enjoy each other within socially acceptable limits. The needs for peer-group activities should be complemented by opportunities for privacy and availability of a "place" that the adolescent can call his own. It is own impression that rooms for one or several adolescents are preferable to open wards.

It is obvious that the hospitalized adolescent has suffered severe deprivation in group life. He has been unable to belong to a group; his past history is replete with failures and rejections. Individual therapy that merely makes one-to-one relationships tolerable cannot replace satisfactory functioning in the group. Here the hospital can make an impressive contribution by providing a variety of groups to which the adolescent can relate, even to the point of manufacturing groups suited to his needs; too, the staff can help him along every step of his attempts to become a full-fledged participant in adolescent culture. Our impression is that the setting we have described, allowing for the formation of small adolescent groups within a larger adult society, was especially well-adapted to these purposes. The presence of the adults was felt chiefly as a stabilizing influence by the adolescents, who appeared to respond to the age and maturity of the adult patients rather than to their individual illnesses.

Group life not only supports the adolescents, but also provides the individual adolescent with mirror images for his problem. Sharing rebellious urges aids in their sublimation and facilitates emancipation. The hospital group situation, for example, makes it possible to act out in part the conflict with authority through the setting-up and overthrow of group leaders. It teaches responsibility in that each adolescent must contribute something to help the group remain alive; no one is supposed to destroy its overall goals or its "fun." Thus, role-testing, experimentation with being this or that person, all before a ready-made responsive audience, is now possible. The formation and break-up of companionships and alliances, the playing with attitudes toward authority and peers, all on a less serious and less deep plane than the level of his basic problems, yet very symbolic, meaningful, and potentially therapeutic, now can be acted out. Moreover, the context is usually one that provides pleasures and rewards of being with others.

This group process cannot be left to chance, nor does it necessarily happen to every hospitalized adolescent simply as a result of proximity to groups. It is an active process in which sensitive experts in group relations can play a great role of interpreting, interacting, or subtly directing the group experience. This expertise cannot be automatically transferred from individual to group therapy, but has to be learned and developed by special study and clinical experience with group life. Skill in individual relations is probably a necessary precondition, but it is not by itself the full condition for adequacy in group therapy.

We must recognize that there are definite shortcomings in a hospital program, no matter how successful it may be. The main problem is lack of permanence of group membership; when the adolescent is discharged he must seek another, more definitive, healthier group in the community. A great deal of effort and perhaps suffering has finally won him a place in ward society, but outside he has to evolve all over again. In the favorable case hope and confidence are higher from having already achieved success.

Our psychiatric follow-up showed that 53 per cent of our Cohort was still without any real peer relationships in the year following discharge. It is clear, therefore, that intensive follow-up and continued community care are necessary parts of a total integrated treatment program. Community care is still the more neglected aspect which in the future will require much experience and study.

The natural community group will not be so responsive to the adolescent's needs as was the hospital community; he will have to adapt to reality as given. However, in cases where clinically indicated, special groups created as stepping stones for shaky patients would be a great advantage. Prevention-of-hospitalization-clubs, somewhat along the lines of Alcoholics Anonymous, halfway residences, and socialization centers, stimulated and supervised by hospital staff, need to be developed. This will not only help to insure success in doubtful cases but will go a long way toward preventing relapse and rehospitalization.

INTELLECTUAL MASTERY: SCHOOL

The typical hospitalized adolescent has had severely traumatic experiences in his school career and may have been rejected by school administration. As a consequence he is blocked in his intellectual development, falls behind his contemporaries, and the process of learning itself becomes an area of anxiety. His rejection by school closes off important therapeutic avenues related to mastery of his difficulties with his peers, resolution of inner conflicts, and discovery of a meaningful role in society. At this age, failure in school is a failure in life. We have seen in this study that after treatment many adolescents are again able to indulge that consuming curiosity that characterized them in health.

The process of dealing with inhibited intellectual life is a task not only for the psychotherapist, but also for specifically trained educators assisted by a flexible and varied classroom program. The program should be prepared to offer new challenges to fit the adolescent's intellectual level rather than only his last school grade. It should offer tangible rewards for accomplishments similar to those which prevail in schools outside—promotions, scholarships, and opportunities for advanced study. Especially important is the transferability of credits from sheltered schools to community schools, as was available in this setting.

VOCATIONAL MASTERY: WORK

The further achievement of a sense of identity requires the adolescent to learn an occupation and obtain a job in the workaday world. The hospital must recognize the need for his progress in the occupational sphere and provisions should be made for a multifaceted occupational-rehabilitation program.

What are the requirements of a good occupational-rehabilitation program? First, the philosophy that useful work and occupational self-sufficiency are important goals in life, that work not only facilitates emotional stability, but is also a source of happiness and satisfaction. Work gives the adolescent status in the world of the adult responsibility as well as a necessary bulwark against boredom and apathy. There is clearly something therapeutic in the daily mobilization and expenditure of energy in a useful task.

Too often the view is held that because patients are ill or the State pays their way, there is no obligation to work or earn. To institutionalize the philosophy that work is therapeutic requires special effort not only on the part of the administration, but on the part of professionals and ward personnel as well.

A second principle is that work must fit the interests and capabilities of the patient; it must be tailored to his needs and abilities at the time, changing as he changes with age, training, and increasing ability and experience. This means a broad, flexible program planned for immediate and long-range goals. The hospital must provide an analysis of patients' interests and abilities, an occupational diagnosis, job counselling, job training, good work environment with therapeutically sophisticated work supervisors, and a routine of work activities patterned as closely as possible on conditions outside. Some of the many elements required at the practical level are trained rehabilitation and work-coordinators to complement the occupational therapists; a variety of workshops under supervisors who are a true part of the rehabilitation program receiving instruction and guidance themselves; systematic re-examination and re-evaluation of work performance for change or reassignment; and collaboration and coordination with professionals concerned with other aspects of the patient's life. An employment office, a job finding service, and follow-up are necessary elements. All this will develop around individual and group counselling aimed at resolving work tensions and impasses at both the psychological and social level, often with family participation. The reader will appreciate that this is a tall order for most hospitals.

There are also considerations related to the age of the patient. For those under sixteen, the program will mostly be concerned with discussions and educational sessions that orient the adolescent to the realities of the world of work; however, after sixteen years of age the adolescent often will be able to enter more directly into the task of becoming an independent worker and earner. It must also be stated that a top level rehabilitation program will require collaboration of the hospital with agencies outside, State rehabilitation programs, sheltered workshops and the like.

DEVELOPMENT OF A PHILOSOPHY OF LIFE

Adolescence is a formative period during which, in addition to the above tasks, the individual begins to approach problems as old as man, unsolved larger issues toward which we must all adopt some attitude. These have to do with ethics, morality, religion, and the choice between various codes of behavior. What is honor, friendship, loyalty, and responsibility toward others as opposed to satisfaction of narcissistic needs alone? What is proper conduct with respect to the opposite sex? What sort of family will one establish in the future? These and a host of other questions about life sooner or later concern the adolescent, though often not explicitly stated by him.

Many youths on the wards of the MMHC before admission were in such severe conflict between the sexual drives and parental opposition to masturbation, for example, that they had never been able to establish mutual confidence with another person. In other cases, values were so grossly distorted by a mentally-ill parent in the home that the hospitalized adolescent had no idea about group sports, never having been allowed to participate in athletics by a fearful mother. Others had never attended a party or a dance because dancing was "sinful." Some of the hospitalized adolescents had been taught not to trust neighbors, and their parents were continually moving from one residence to another. Some fathers refused to allow teenage children to go to church, to have spending money, or to make purchases.

On the wards of the MMHC there was, as we have observed, a great deal of interaction between the adolescent patients and their peers—whether "court cases," student nurses, college-student attendants, or medical students. For many of the severely withdrawn boys, the long talks with the student nurse assigned to them, dancing with female patients and female students, and mixed socializing in the day hall were new experiences. The young attendant

strumming his guitar, the young resident psychiatrist sitting patiently by the hour waiting for the adolescent to say just *one*
friendly word, were new and slightly incredible happenings. These
experiences however, often opened up the possibility of a new view
of life.

In an ideal environment, values important to the adolescent—
caring, honesty, patience, dedication to the welfare of others—can
be exemplified in the ward society. In sports he develops new attitudes toward winning and losing. He learns to try his best for the
sake of the team even if victory is denied. College students as
attendants and recreational leaders who are athletically inclined
can play a very important role for adolescent patients in this respect. The "good sport" concept can become the rudiment of
morality and eventual ethical practice of the adult.

In the strictly religious sphere, we have found that the basic
attitudes expressed by the adolescent are primarily the product of
his sickness. If "God is the father," then, during the adolescent's
authority rebellion he will reject religion, especially the religion of
his father, albeit in an ambivalent and guilty fashion. As authority
problems begin to be solved, the youngster will adopt a softer
attitude toward religion and what it can offer.

We have found that theological students can be very effective in
helping adolescent patients develop a philosophy of life.[12] When
the adolescent patient returned home and told his parents that the
priest or minister considered it important for him to open a bank
account, or to decide how to spend his own money earned through
work, the parents were impressed. Often the clergy were regarded
as more impartial members of the community than psychiatrists or
other hospital employees. Thus, theological students were great
assets in helping adolescent patients unlearn bizarre cultural values
adopted from their parents.

THE IDEAL ENVIRONMENT

The establishment of an adolescent service with both inpatient
and community branches which tries to adapt a complex network
of therapeutic activities to the individual needs of a number of ado-

---

[12] Luzzi, M., and Glasser, B. A.; Adolescent patients join the neighborhood
youth corps, Hosp. & Commu. Psychiat. 172-175, 1966.

lescents requires leadership, coordination, intensive communication among responsible heads of departments, professionals and ward workers, and flexibility to suit the changing demands of the individual patients. Needless to say, this calls for high sophistication on the part of the administration and puts a considerable burden upon student psychiatrists, who, fresh out of internship, are put in charge of wards with all their complicated programs. Ward personnel, in turn, often with many years of experience in dealing with psychotic patients, must try to fulfill the dual role of acknowledging the young doctor as leader and at the same time serving as his instructor. Harmonious personal relationships among staff workers depend largely on the degree of mutual respect between them, and this in turn reflects the interest in fostering good morale demonstrated by leaders. In addition to the many specific suggestions we have made as to setting, it is well to bear in mind the wisdom of the U.N. Expert Committee that concerned itself with factors determining therapeutic success in different treatment organizations:

"The most important single factor in the efficacy of the treatment given in a mental hospital appears to the committee to be an intangible element which can only be described as its atmosphere. . . . As in the community at large, one of the characteristic aspects of the psychiatric hospital is the type of relationship between people that are to be found within it. The nature of the relationships between the medical director and his staff will be reflected in the relationship between the psychiatric staff and the nurses, and finally in the relationship not only between the nurses and the patients, but between the patients themselves."[13]

---

[13] Expert Committee on Mental Health, Third Report, World Health Organization, Technical Report Series No. 73, Geneva, 1953 pp. 17-18.

PART VII

Epilogue

Five or more years have passed since our Cohort left the sheltering environment of the MMHC. Have the patients improved or deteriorated? How have they adapted? Have they managed to survive in the world outside?

CHAPTER 17

Five Years Later—The Adolescent Patients as Young Adults

It is now possible to present some results of a five-year follow-up study of the Cohort. Information is available concerning thirty of the forty-six patients for whom a five-year interval since discharge has elapsed. Thirteen of the forty-six could not be located, two refused to be interviewed, and one died in an automobile accident.

These patients, now age twenty to twenty-four, are no longer considered by society as adolescents but rather as young adults. Does the change of status with the passing of years affect the level of adaptation of individuals who were regarded as very sick five years ago?

There are only a few published long-term follow-up studies of hospitalized adolescents, only one of which followed patients five years or more after discharge. This study, by Masterson,[14,15] showed

Based on work by Libby Herrera

[14] Masterson, J. F.: Prognosis in adolescent disorders. Amer. J. Psychiat. 114: 1097, 1958.
[15] Masterson, J. F.: Prognosis in adolescent disorders—Schizophrenia. J. Nerv. Ment. Dis. 124: 219, 1956.

a high rate of improvement at time of discharge from the hospital. The improvement tended to be maintained in most of the neurotic patients, but there was a high rate of deterioration in the sicker patients, especially those with a diagnosis of schizophrenia.

METHOD OF STUDY

The five-year follow-up study here discussed was undertaken as a sequel to the six-month social service and one-year psychiatric follow-up studies of the Cohort (Chapters 12 and 13). Insofar as was practicable, comparable information was sought and the same criteria for rating were applied.

All contacts, as well as all ratings, were made by one research social worker who, to eliminate bias, had read neither the patients' records nor previous follow-up material prior to interviewing or rating. Patients were easily reassured during interviews that any ignorance on the part of the interviewer about family constellation, etc. was an intended aspect of the research plan. All patients were seen no sooner than five and no later than five and one-quarter years from the time of discharge from their first admission to MMHC.

Each patient was sent a letter on hospital stationery requesting that he come to the MMHC for an interview of approximately one hour to discuss his current life situation as a way of cooperating in a research project aimed at improving services to adolescent patients. Of the thirty patients who could be located, twelve had moved since their last contact with the hospital, rarely leaving forwarding addresses, so that numerous letters and telephone calls were required even to secure a correct address. Patients were also frequently unreliable about arranging for and keeping appointments; only three returned the stamped, addressed post-cards included in each letter on which they were asked to note confirmation of their appointment or to suggest an alternate time. One patient made three two-hour bus trips at times other than those agreed upon for appointments before he was able to come at a time when he could be seen.

Only when patients were unavailable or clearly unreliable was an attempt made to contact related persons or agencies. The principal informants in nineteen cases were the patients themselves—fifteen in office interviews, two in their homes, and two in mental institutions. The wish of some patients to have no personal contact with the hospital was respected and, other than ascertaining that they had received the letter requesting an appointment, no pressure was brought to bear. Parents, usually interviewed by telephone, were the principal sources of information in eight cases. A court probation officer, a social worker, and a psychiatrist, respectively, were the main sources of information in three others. Whenever it seemed advisable, a combination of sources was consulted.

Almost without exception, parents and patients who were actually interviewed welcomed the opportunity to talk with someone. Several used the occasion of coming into the hospital to look up former acquaintances on the staff with the same nostalgic overtones of someone returning to visit a beloved alma mater. In four instances, patients currently in psychotherapy asked their therapists to approach the research social worker first to satisfy their anxieties as to the real purpose of the interview.

Although the interviewer limited her own responses exclusively to those directed toward information-gathering during the semiformal research interview, she spent a few minutes at the end on therapeutic questions. Four patients were urged to resume psychotherapy. Another patient was given help in clarifying his draft status while for still another, several telephone calls were made in an effort to involve him in some community social activity. Many patients had questions and comments about the research project. Three voiced relief as they left that it had not been as difficult to come as they had thought it would be. Before leaving patients were also told that some member of the research staff might be contacting them again in another five years.

As in the other follow-up studies, information about current level of functioning was sought in the three specific areas of family, social, and school-work adjustment. The following specific questions within each of these areas were covered during the course of the interview.

Family Relationships:

Who was living within the home? How did patient get along with family members? Description of interaction with various household members and description of a typical day.

Social Relationships:

Did patient have friends? Of the same or opposite sex? One? or how many? A description of peer relationships, hobbies, recreational pursuits, community activities, etc.

School and/or Work Adjustment:

A description of the study or work program, especially in terms of emotional, intellectual involvement. How much time and effort is required? Patient's opinion of and reaction to these requirements.

Adjustment in each of these three areas was rated as being *Good, Fair,* or *Poor* according to the criteria described in the psychiatric follow-up study (Chapter 13).

A fourth rating made was overall level of functioning (Chapter 12). In this category the ratings in the three specific areas outlined above were considered in addition to such questions as:

How did the patient present himself? Physical appearance and behavior during the interview? Physical health, energy level, and mood? Patient's own assessment of his current mental status? What was patient's reaction to coming for the interview and how did he react with interviewer?

Taken into account when making this rating was stability of functioning; for example, if it was "Good" at the moment but looked especially vulnerable or rigidly circumscribed it was rated as being only "Fair."

Finally a rating of improvement was made: The patient's current level of functioning was compared with his functioning described under the heading of "chief complaint" in his original admission records, and he was rated as being *Improved, Same,* or *Worse.*

RESULTS

Considering their average age of over twenty-two years, the Cohort appeared to be atypical in terms of marital status, living arrangements, education, and vocation. Of the thirty patients, all had remained single except for two girls who were married and living with their husbands. Fourteen of the thirty patients were still living with their parents, one was living alone at home since his mother's death, one lived with grandparents in preference to living with parents, seven lived in apartments, usually alone, and four were in mental hospitals. Only one was away in college.

Table XXII indicates how the Cohort was rated in the four areas of family, social, and school-work adjustment, and overall functioning five years after discharge. There were fewer patients rated *Poor* in family relationships than in the other areas. This area was apparently the most successful for the group in terms of adjustment. However, the material obtained in the interviews strongly suggests that families were tolerating considerable psychopathology, frequently altering their own patterns to meet the patients' needs and thus mask severe difficulties.

Table XXIII shows significant reduction in the number of poor family relationships from the time of the first follow-up. Part of this movement runs parallel to the overall improvement of patients; however, it does not occur so strongly in the other areas of adjustment and may give further credence to the argument that it is the family that adjusts to the sick person rather than he to the family.

TABLE XXII

Five-year Follow-up Adjustment Ratings

	Overall Adjustment	Family Adjustment	Social Adjustment	School-work Adjustment
Good	7	14	4	15
Fair	15	12	10	4
Poor	8	3	16	11
Total	30	29°	30	30

° No immediate family living, in one case.

TABLE XXIII

Family Adjustment in Three Follow-up Studies

	Good	Fair	Poor	Total
Six months	8	6	16	30
One year	7	8	10	25°
Five years	14	12	3	29†

° No information on five patients.
† Family no longer living, in one case.

Almost without exception, patients did very poorly in the area of social relationships in the five year evaluations (Table XXIV). This

TABLE XXIV

Social Adjustment in Three Follow-up Studies

	Good	Fair	Poor	Total
Six months	11	7	12	30
One year	4	7	14	25*
Five years	4	10	16	30

* No information on five of these patients.

adjustment was not too different from that seen at one year, but markedly worse than that seen at six months. Perhaps at the six-month evaluation, patients were still coasting with the impetus of pressure from various hospital elements but subsequently reverted to their strong tendencies toward social seclusion, for secluded many of them certainly were at the five-year follow-up. Even patients with otherwise very good adjustment showed severe problems in this, clearly the most difficult area of adjustment. In fact some of the relatively successful patients appeared to have consciously focused their interest on other areas to the exclusion of any but the most superficial social contacts, thus insulating themselves from what they seemed to be an area of inevitable failure. This phenomenon provides an excellent example of how possibly unsolvable inadequacies can be denied and compensated for by developing alternative areas of strength.

Among the Cohort, there was a striking paucity of commitment to or communication with the community. These patients were totally uninvolved with social resources with the exception of nine who attended church, all but one sporadically and under family pressure. This was predictable because of their difficulty in forming relationships. However, it also poses the question as to how the community might more effectively meet its obligation to these isolated people who form an increasing proportion of our society.

Considering their intellectual and socio-economic assets, the average educational and vocational achievement level of the Cohort five years after discharge was very poor. None of the group had completed college; twelve had never completed high school. Table XXV shows school-work adjustment at the time of each of the three fol-

TABLE XXV

School-Work Adjustment in Three Follow-up Studies

	Good	Fair	Poor	Total
Six months	10	3	17	30
One year	11		14	25*
Five years	15	4	11	30

* No information on five of these patients.

low-up studies. There appeared to be slight improvement over the years. However, over one-third of the Cohort was still doing poorly, which means being idle—both educationally and vocationally. Of the nineteen who were involved in work or study, the distribution was as follows:

Full-time work 10
Full schedule college 2
Full college plus part-time work 2
Full-time work plus part-time college 2
Part-time work and college 2
Part-time work 1

Total 19

The type of work in which patients were involved tended to be unskilled or semiskilled: garbage collector, waitress, hospital orderly, cashier in a grocery store, etc. Only three had attained more sophisticated levels of employment such as secretarial work. One had found, with a combination of good luck and merit, an employer who was grooming him for a position as foreman in a construction firm, giving him time and encouragement to attend college classes related to that field.

In terms of overall level of functioning, seven patients were rated *Good*, fifteen *Fair*, and eight *Poor*. Quite significantly, and contrary to expectations based on the findings of other studies, there was improvement in the rating of overall level of functioning from the six-month follow-up study to the five-year follow-up study in these thirty patients (Table XXVI). Whereas at six months only one patient was rated as having a *Good* overall level of functioning, at five years there were seven patients in that category. Some of the patients had received a considerable amount of psychotherapy since discharge from the hospital, but there was no significant relation-

TABLE XXVI

Overall Level of Functioning Ratings in Sixth-Month and Five-Year Follow-up Studies

	Good	Fair	Poor
Six months	1	11	18
Five years	7	15	8

ship between amount of therapy and level of functioning five years after discharge.

The majority of the patients interviewed (73 per cent) were rated as *Improved* since original admission at the five-year follow-up study. Table XXVII shows how this rating of change compares with that seen for the same thirty patients in the two earlier follow-ups. Only one patient was found to be *Worse* since admission, as compared with seven and four in the first two studies.

Table XXVIII compares the overall improvement ratings for each patient at six months and at five years after discharge. Improvement for the large number of patients has remained steady. The group rated *Worse* at six months did surprisingly well: five of the seven were rated *Improved* in the five-year follow-up. However, five patients who showed symptomatic improvement at six months drifted back to their pre-hospitalization status.

From Table XXIX (relationship between overall improvement at one year and five years), it is clear that most patients considered *Improved* at one year were still *Improved* five years after discharge. Eight of the Cohort who were unimproved at the time of the one year follow-up, at five years were judged to be better than at the

TABLE XXVII

Improvement in Patients Since Time of Admission

	Improved	No Change	Worse	Total
Six months social work follow-up	17	6	7	30
One year psychiatric follow-up	15	9	4	28*
Five year follow-up	22	7	1	30

* No information on two of the thirty patients included in the five-year follow-up.

time of admission. Four patients, however, had regressed from *Improved* at one year, to *Same* five years after discharge.

Many patients who were rated *Same* had unfortunately become chronically ineffectual, marginally adjusted at best, unemployed, and with little life outside their families.

Table XXX shows the relationship of improvement ratings and rating of overall level of functioning in the five-year follow-up study. Although patients who showed improvement also tended to have better level of functioning, the table indicates that even in the "Improved" group, level of functioning was more frequently *Fair* than *Good*.

TABLE XXVIII

Relationship between Overall Improvement
at Six Months and Five Years

Six-month Follow-up Study	Five-year Follow-up Study			
	Improved	No Change	Worse	Total
Improved	12	5		17
No Change	5	1		6
Worse	5	1	1	7
Total	22	7	1	30

TABLE XXIX

Relationship between Overall Improvement
at One Year and Five Years

One Year Follow-up Study	Five-year Follow-up Study			
	Improved	No Change	Worse	Total
Improved	11*	4		15
No Change	8	1		9
Worse	1	2	1	4
Total	22	7	1	30

* Two of the Cohort improved in five year follow-up were not included in one-year follow-up.

TABLE XXX

*Overall Level of Functioning and its Relationship
to Improvement Rating*

Five-year Follow-up Over-all Level of Functioning	Change Since Admission		
	Improved	No Change	Worse
Good	7	0	0
Fair	14	1	0
Poor	1	6	1
Total	22	7	1

CASE STUDIES—FIVE YEARS AFTER DISCHARGE

Patrick: Patrick is now twenty-four years old. Since graduating from high school, Patrick has changed jobs several times. At present he is working in the mail room of a new large office building. However, he still talks of broadcasting as his ultimate goal. He and his mother own a car jointly and drive to work together while his father, who because of several heart attacks in the past years requires a sedentary job, goes to work, when he does work, by streetcar. The family has continued to move every other year and is presently planning another move. Patrick has a barren social life—almost completely devoid of any relationships outside his mother and father. He told the interviewer that it is his intention never to marry. During the interview he chain-smoked and chewed on his fingernails. He has had no therapy since discharge and feels he has no need for any despite occasional periods of depression.

Patrick's life pattern seems to be settling into one of a seriously constricted, "odd ball," marginal person.

Linda: Linda is now twenty-two. After two years at home during which time she neither worked nor attended school, Linda was recently rehospitalized. She is currently on the violent ward at a state hospital, under heavy sedation, taking Trilafon and Artane. She is not receiving any psychotherapy. Her present psychotic episode was precipitated, according to the hospital social worker, by her reading in the newspapers about the killing of twelve student nurses in Chicago. Linda's mother visits her weekly, and the family is willing to have her home on weekend visits. This girl seems to be settling into a life pattern of chronic patienthood. The continuing support by her family might perhaps be considered a hopeful feature; nonetheless, at present Linda shows little evidence of ability to function in any role other than that of a chronic schizophrenic patient.

DISCUSSION

As a group our Cohort showed a significant tendency toward improvement at the time of the five-year follow-up study. However, the unfortunate fact remains that most of the thirty patients evaluated were still seriously handicapped by mental disorder. None were really free of symptoms; three who were functioning quite well nevertheless voiced fears concerning the precariousness of their adjustment. As a group they were performing and contributing to society on a level which fell far short of normal expectations.

It is a sobering fact that in this group, psychotherapy, during hospitalization or afterwards, was not associated with any striking gains. Some of the patients were still in therapy at the time of follow-up, and further gains are possible. It is also possible that therapy rescued a few who otherwise would have fared much worse. Nonetheless, the data from the group as a whole supplied little evidence for this.

The very moderate but definite gradual improvement in the group over the years is a process that, in our opinion, has two major components. First is the gradual adjustment of the adolescent patient to his environment or vice versa: this mutual process often took considerable time and resulted in a situation that allowed the patient to function relatively successfully, at school and work, but at the cost of avoiding certain painful areas, usually social intercourse. Secondly, the patients were no longer adolescents at the time of the five-year follow-up, and this in itself appears to make a considerable difference in that the period of turmoil, increased sexual and aggressive drive, and rebellion is for the most part over. We cannot estimate to what extent we are looking at a reduction in the strength of instinctual drive after adolescence and to what extent we are seeing chiefly an attempt to meet social pressures and expectations which are very different for a twenty-two-year-old than for a sixteen-year-old. In any case, the fact is that these young men and women are better adjusted to the world than they have been, especially in terms of family relationships and school or work activities.

Index